D1414036

Mental Health Education
in the
New Medical Schools

Donald G. Langsley
John F. McDermott, Jr.
Allen J. Enelow
Editors

Foreword by C. H. Hardin Branch

Mental Health Education
in the
New Medical Schools

 Jossey-Bass Publishers

San Francisco • Washington • London • 1973

MENTAL HEALTH EDUCATION IN THE NEW MEDICAL SCHOOLS
*Donald G. Langsley, John F. McDermott, Jr.,
and Allen J. Enelow, Editors*

Copyright © 1973 by Jossey-Bass, Inc., Publishers
615 Montgomery Street
San Francisco, California 94111

and

Jossey-Bass Limited
3 Henrietta Street
London WC2E 8LU

Copyright under International, Pan American, and
Universal Copyright Conventions. All rights
reserved. No part of this book may be reproduced
in any form—except for brief quotation (not to
exceed 1,000 words) in a review or professional
work—without permission in writing from the publisher.

Library of Congress Catalogue Card Number LC 73-48

International Standard Book Number ISBN 0-87589-167-5

Manufactured in the United States of America

JACKET DESIGN BY WILLI BAUM

FIRST EDITION

Code 7312

The Jossey-Bass
Behavioral Science Series

General Editors

WILLIAM E. HENRY, *University of Chicago*

NEVITT SANFORD, *Wright Institute, Berkeley*

Foreword

This seems to be a propitious time for a new book on psychiatric education. For the obsessively anniversary-minded, we are two decades away from the famous Ithaca conferences of 1951–1952. For the person tuned to current concepts of academic responsibility, the time is ripe for considering social and community concepts as they are anticipated in medical education which prepares physicians to meet newly recognized needs. We have had men to match our mountains; we need now teams psychologically sophisticated enough to match our technologies. What profits a man if he gains a heart or a kidney and loses his soul? How can we measure health and disease in the light of changing values and social revolutions? If health, for example, means the ability to manipulate the welfare structure gracefully and skillfully, what happens to the work ethic of the therapist who would regard this skill as parasitism?

At any rate, there is presently a need to reevaluate medical education and especially psychiatric education. Psychiatry seems destined to operate in the area of the unsolved problems. Those illnesses for which we have developed crisp, definitive treatments have dropped back into the general pool of medicine. We are left with the social-economic-medical problems for which the rest of medicine has no answers and, in fact, little welcome.

The Airlie House Conference was a courageous attempt to deal with the vast array of problems of community psychiatric needs, medical school administration, changing concepts of teaching-learning for medical students, and even the phantasmagoria of financing education in an age when other, more atavistic enterprises seem to have the ascendancy. The planners wisely called on students and residents for answers. They may not have answers but they have not, to paraphrase James Branch Cabell, mastered that invaluable gesture known as the shrug; their contributions were thoughtful and worthwhile. They can, and do, twist the tails of such sacred cows as the department and even the college structure in the universities. And any progress to be made will come from these new medical schools or these new departments in old medical schools. The rest of us will profit from their venturesomeness.

The meeting—I am, of course, judging from the report; I regret that I could not share personally in the activities, although I am flattered to have been consulted in the planning stage—did not entirely desert the past, nor did the past entirely desert it. John Romano's comments sounded as mellifluous and scholarly as those which enriched the Ithaca conferences, and Robert Stubblefield and Walter Barton could and did provide broad perspectives against which experimental ventures in conceptualization, instructional methods, and evaluation stand out in bright relief.

Some themes inevitably recur. The role of psychoanalysis is discussed, but there seems to be tacit agreement that its importance lies in the viability of some elements of the theory and its usefulness in training. Several participants stated that as a therapeutic tool it has little value for the vast mass of emotional ills. Also there were various discussions about the need for departmental and medical school reorganizations to avoid the congealing effect of standard administrative practices. I am not clear as to how the conference felt this reorganization should be done. There is little usefulness in modifying the departmental structure if the power still resides in an executive committee composed of department heads. And unless funds can be made really interdepartmental, each academic bowerbird will continue to guard the brightly colored pebbles in its own nest.

The number of medical school departments which deal with "basic" aspects of the behavioral sciences has increased considerably. Oregon, the University of Southern California, Johns Hopkins, Oklahoma, Maryland, Michigan State, and others have developed departments with various labels and various spheres of influence in the medical school picture. Some of the new department chairmen (Arnold Mandell comes to mind as one example) have been very outspoken in their desire to develop separate departments for clinical and basic psychiatry—the sort of arrangement we oldsters attempted to encompass under one chairmanship. It will take time to determine whether this dichotomy is useful.

A very refreshing aspect of this conference was the consideration of the economic aspects of medical and psychiatric care as these relate to the training of physicians. We have long been aware of some of these problems, but we continue to have the rows of wooden benches in our outpatient clinics, the failure to provide minimum human dignity in our wards, the unrealistic and humiliating hospital procedures which distinguish between the haves and the have-nots. Both the patients and the students have straightened us out on these matters, and medical education is better for it.

It is heartening to see, in a conference of this sort, some consideration given—from the *teaching* aspect, mind you—to health insurance, prepaid medical care, and the HMO concept. The medical care constellations dominated by the medical schools might just possibly be in a position to take the lead in these matters, although they have not yet demonstrated this leadership, and it is highly unlikely organized medicine will desert its entrenched conservatism. But, as Barton pointed out, there is hope that such experiments as the United Auto Workers benefit plan will continue to modify the national health insurance picture, and if departments of psychiatry can get politicians and insurance carriers to look at the actuarial data thus generated, perhaps economic improvements in the delivery of health care services will result. Coverage for mental illnesses can well lead to better coverage for all the multifaceted illness problems.

Unfortunately prepaid medical care plans have not been

better incorporated into the medical school picture, although there were suggestions in the conference that Kaiser Permanente plans might be useful models. From a purely nostalgic point of view, I am sorry that the Ross-Loos Medical Group in Los Angeles has not received more recognition as a pioneer in this field. In some form, prepaid medical care systems may turn out to provide reasonable answers to medical economic problems while offering settings in which medical education can optimally take place.

The fundamental contribution of the conference, however, was the recognition of the shift from the unitary concept of medical care to the multiplex concept and the recognition of the need for different training to accomplish this goal. The pattern of one patient, one disease, one therapist in one facility has been replaced by a treatment situation in which the patient should often be regarded simply as a delegate representing the pathology in his district (his family and the neighborhood). His treatment is then necessarily carried out by a treatment complex and in a range of facilities which may extend geographically far beyond any one location. Adequate and effective manipulation of this process demands a different sophistication from that found in the traditional medical school curriculum, and the conference has noted and developed this fact.

All in all, *Mental Health Education in the New Medical Schools* has many useful elements, not the least of which are the detailed descriptions of the various programs in the new schools and an outline of available teaching aids. As Romano points out, many conferences on psychiatric education have produced "sizable and sometimes readable reports." This document is both sizable and readable and in addition is informative. The effect of this enterprise to which Donald Langsley, Allen Enelow, and John McDermott have contributed so much in energy, dedication, and their own experiences should be far-reaching and lasting. It will be to their credit if this book spawns a new breed of psychiatric educators.

January 1973   C. H. HARDIN BRANCH
                                                  Program Chief
                                                  Santa Barbara County
                                                  Mental Health Service

Preface

Among the many problems facing mental health professionals today, one of the most pressing is education. Every educator, whether a medical school faculty member, a residency training director, or a teacher in a graduate education program, is asking himself to whom should he direct his education, and for what. Psychiatry might be said, with justice, to be experiencing an identity crisis, reflected in the most burning issues of psychiatry education.

No one is sure what the role of the psychiatrist will be in another generation. Students and residents ask, "What does the psychiatrist do that is medical? Why have an M.D. degree?" The other mental health professions, social work, psychiatric nursing, psychology, are assuming more and more of the once-traditional prerogatives of the psychiatrist and asking the same questions. The designation of the psychiatrist as captain of the mental health team no longer goes undisputed. Perhaps the community mental health movement, as much or more than any other one factor, has highlighted these issues. Especially in areas with a low concentration of psychiatric manpower, one is likely to find a social worker or psychologist as director of a community mental health center.

In undergraduate psychiatry education, similar questions are being asked. Should psychiatrist teachers direct their efforts to the future nonpsychiatrist, identifying core skills and knowledge he will need in his practice of medicine, or continue to teach him about the specialty of psychiatry? How much of what is done by the psychiatrist could be done by the family doctor or general internist if he were trained and motivated to do it? The area of preclinical psychiatry, the introduction of which into the curriculum was a hard-fought and relatively recently won battle by psychiatrists to wrest preclinical curriculum time from the basic scientists, is now in dispute. Should this training be the responsibility of psychiatry or be given to a department of behavioral science?

And, of course, within psychiatry itself, the question is where are we going and what will our role be? Will psychiatry move more and more into public programs? Will there continue to be a full-time M.D. psychotherapist? And as new medical schools develop without university hospitals, a growing trend, where will our locus of training activities be found?

Regardless of what stand a given educator takes on these issues, still other problems face him. Blocks of time and topic-oriented curricula are now under heavy fire. Critics of these traditional approaches to planning training programs are proposing that behavioral objectives for learners must be designed and keyed to assessments of learner progress at all educational levels—undergraduate, residency, and continuing education. With increasing frequency, one hears that the traditional programs make time a constant and quality of product (the graduate) a variable and that this relation should be altered so that time is the variable and quality becomes a constant. Another proposal is for integrated training programs: integration of subject matter as well as integration of students of different professions or disciplines studying the same material. Still another proposal stems from the apparently growing public demand for periodic recertification or relicensure.

Together with all medical educators and health professional educators we are beginning to question the previously accepted concept that a professional degree, clinical training, and clinical experience are adequate qualifications for designing and conducting training programs. Such a background usually does not include learning how to teach and how to facilitate learning. The fact that a number of medical schools have added divisions or offices of medical education since 1960 reflects increasing concern with this issue. Medical educators are taking a close look at peer-group instruction and self-instruction as possible means to facilitate learning and make the most efficient use of instructor time.

The new medical schools have an excellent opportunity to experiment with new models because of the absence of those constraints that stem from vested interests and traditional practices; they can examine all these and related issues and construct programs that can try to produce solutions to the dilemmas we now face. This is a unique time in the history of medical education. Twenty-eight schools are now in the process of formation in various stages from the drawing board to the point of graduating the first class.

We, as a committee of the American Association of Chairmen of Departments of Psychiatry, proposed that the association sponsor a three-day retreat meeting of representatives of departments of psychiatry in new medical schools to examine the vital issues confronting psychiatry as they are reflected in these new schools. New medical schools were defined as all schools with provisional accreditation by the American Medical Association (AMA) and the Association of American Medical Colleges (AAMC) or as listed by AMA–AAMC as in the process of formation. Many schools which are relatively new were therefore not included because they had graduated at least one class and had full accreditation. To add balance, resource people were invited. These included new chairmen of psychiatry in existing older medical schools and the speakers. The conference was held at Airlie House in Warrenton, Virginia, February 21–23, 1972, and was supported by a grant from the National Institute of Mental Health #MH 11901-03 S1.

The issues we proposed to examine at that conference and which are the substance of *Mental Health Education in the New Medical Schools* were these: Medical curricula are now including more material and giving more attention to broadening medical students' knowledge and understanding of human behavior. It is now commonly recognized that the psychosocial factors affecting individuals and communities have an important role in incidence and prevalence of disease and affect the success of attempts to provide health care. How then can we provide learning experiences that will give students an appropriate knowledge base and an appreciation of the importance of understanding human behavior, both individual and group? Does the inclusion in the curriculum of behavioral science, a term which is used rather loosely and most often refers to the social sciences, provide this understanding? Or will students turn away from behavioral science, as they often do from the basic biological sciences? Is behavioral science best taught by psychiatry, by a separate department of behavioral science, or by individuals from departments of psychology, sociology, and social anthropology?

Can we provide learning experiences in realistic practice settings rather than in classrooms, in the instance of behavioral science, or in university hospitals, in the instance of clinical sciences? Closely related is the issue of teaching students in community hospitals. Few, if any, new university hospitals are planned. Most of the new medical schools will be forced to work in community hospitals, thus raising a whole host of problems with which medical educators have had little experience. Who controls the hospital? How is power shared with the community as a whole and with the privately practicing medical community? How do we ensure that students will have access to patients, will be provided with proper supervision, and will have good role models while protecting the practitioner and his professional relationships with patients?

These questions, which relate to the setting in which we teach, touch on others that reflect the changing picture of health care and the systems designed to provide it. Apparently the national consensus is that access to our present system is difficult for most citizens, and especially those of lower socioeconomic status and members of ethnic minorities. A parallel contention is that access to a system that will help people to achieve and maintain health is a right of all citizens and not a privilege of the affluent. These conclusions cannot help but bring about changes in our health care system. What part is the medical school to play? Should we design and operate model systems? In such systems that improve access, efficiency, and effectiveness are many more nonmedical professionals than physicians. Should we concern ourselves with training only physicians or all members of the health care team? How much effort should we expend on developing the so-called new careers? All these concerns are intimately bound up with the twin social problems of poverty and racism. Here we see health as an issue that cannot be separated from those of housing, nutrition, education, cultural life and recreation, social organization, and the provision of security under equitable laws. But to what extent should medicine in general or psychiatry in particular address itself to these problems? The rapid growth of community mental health programs has brought psychiatry into much greater participation than formerly in seeking solutions to these problems. How should that change be reflected in psychiatry education?

Among the problems we must face is the growing awareness of a need to reexamine how we teach and what we teach. Psychiatry has been accused of being parochial and of helping to produce the schism between it and the rest of medicine. Most psychiatry educators consider the other fields to be at least equally culpable. The characteristic medical curriculum is departmentally organized and provides little integration of the specialties of medicine; thus, the whole patient is rarely considered an appropriate focus. At best, lip service is paid to the concept. Does the existence of the department itself, as an administrative structure, militate against integration? A few new schools have taken away most of the traditional functions of departments and reassigned them to interdisciplinary structures. A most appropriate question, then, for an organization of department chairmen to examine is: are departments necessary? If departments are not as necessary as once thought, what about blocks of time devoted to one specialty or discipline? Integrated teaching would do away with them. But then how do we define the core curriculum?

Many related questions in undergraduate psychiatry, as in all undergraduate as well as graduate medical education, arise as soon as one examines the conventional style of medical education. How long should training be? Is the M.D. degree an end point? Should there be any end point? Many educators are advocating increased elective time. Some medical schools are now proposing a completely elective curriculum. However, if the usual examinations are given and no alternatives to the usual courses, this provision is an empty gesture, as the student must take all the courses in order to pass all the examinations, and to qualify for his degree. Related to the issue of electives is that of multiple tracks. When should the student begin to specialize? Should the future psychiatrist, the future surgeon, and the future internist all have the same course of studies?

One hears more and more about competency-based program sometimes referred to as the mastery model of education. We decided to examine this approach, which consists of providing the learner with a set of instructional objectives stated in behavioral terms, a variety of ways of achieving the objectives, and regularly scheduled assessments of his progress. If this technique is feasible, time could indeed become a variable and the quality of product—the graduate —much more of a constant.

And last, but not the least important by any means, is the question of funding psychiatry education and especially residency training. Psychiatry is becoming increasingly an outpatient specialty with emphasis on indirect services. Since hospital bed occupancy is the key to funding most residency training (the money being generated by daily charges to bed patients), psychiatry has turned to other sources of funding, primarily governmental. However, basic support for psychiatry training from the National Institute of Mental Health is being reduced and may soon be ending. It is no longer possible to rely on hospital charges for bed occupancy to fund psychiatry programs. How will we find alternative sources to replace the diminishing federal funds without taking retrogressive steps in patient care? We can be certain that the question of funding medical education will become increasingly important as our health care system changes.

These were the issues that we met to discuss and explore. The chapters are position papers prepared by resource persons for discussion at the meetings, while the sections entitled "Discussion" reflect the issues that emerged in response. The discussions were recorded, transcribed, and rewritten by us. We hope the results have captured the essence of the exchange.

**Supported by grant MH 11901-03 S1
from the National Institute of Mental Health**

January 1973   DONALD G. LANGSLEY
                                        JOHN F. McDERMOTT, JR.
                                        ALLEN J. ENELOW

Contents

Foreword   ix
     C. H. Hardin Branch

Preface   xiii

Contributors   xxiii

ONE: UNDERGRADUATE PSYCHIATRIC EDUCATION   1

1. Undergraduate Programs: The McMaster
   Experience   3
        C. A. Adsett

2. Behavioral Sciences: Wherefrom, Whether,
   and W(h)ither?   19
        H. L. P. Resnik

Discussion   30

TWO: RESIDENCY TRAINING PROGRAMS   35

3. Goals and Issues in Psychiatric Residency
    Training   37
    Robert L. Stubblefield

4. Training for Community Service   42
    Walter W. Shervington
    Discussion   50

THREE: NEW SETTINGS   57

5. Clinical Settings for Educational Programs   59
    John Romano

6. Planning and Implementing New Strategies   65
    Thomas G. Webster

    Discussion   71

FOUR: PLANNING AND EVALUATION OF TRAINING   77

7. Instructional Objectives and Priorities   79
    Hilliard Jason

8. Evaluating Student Performance   88
    Bryce Templeton

    Discussion   99

FIVE: FUNDING   113

9. Funding Mental Health Services   115
    Claudewell S. Thomas, Henry A. Foley

10. Impact of National Health Insurance   127
    Walter E. Barton

Discussion   139

Epilogue: Prospects for the Seventies   147
        Donald G. Langsley

Appendix A: Program Descriptions of Mental
        Health Education in the New Medical
        Schools   163

Appendix B: Annotated Bibliography on Mental
        Health Education and List of Resources
        for Instructional Aids   230

Bibliography   241

Index   247

Contributors

C. A. ADSETT, *professor of psychiatry, McMaster University Medical Centre, Hamilton, Ontario*

WALTER E. BARTON, *medical director, American Psychiatric Association*

ALLEN J. ENELOW, *chairman, Department of Psychiatry, Pacific Medical Center, and professor of psychiatry, University of the Pacific*

HENRY A. FOLEY, *health economist, Division of Mental Health Service Programs, National Institute of Mental Health*

HILLIARD JASON, *professor and director, Office of Medical Education Research and Development, and professor of psychiatry and of educational psychology, Michigan State University*

DONALD G. LANGSLEY, *professor and chairman, Department of Psychiatry, University of California, Davis, School of Medicine, and director, Sacramento County Mental Health Services*

JOHN F. McDERMOTT, JR., *professor and chairman of psychiatry, University of Hawaii School of Medicine*

H. L. P. RESNIK, *chief, Center for Studies of Suicide Prevention, National Institute of Mental Health*

JOHN ROMANO, *Distinguished University Professor of Psychiatry, University of Rochester School of Medicine and Dentistry*

WALTER W. SHERVINGTON, *chief, Psychiatry Training Branch, National Institute of Mental Health*

ROBERT L. STUBBLEFIELD, *associate director for mental health, Western Interstate Commission for Higher Education*

BRYCE TEMPLETON, *associate director, National Board of Medical Examiners*

CLAUDEWELL S. THOMAS, *director, Division of Mental Health Service Programs, National Institute of Mental Health*

THOMAS G. WEBSTER, *professor and chairman, George Washington University School of Medicine*

Participants in the
Airlie House Conference

New Medical Schools

Brown University (Providence)—BEN W. FEATHER, *chairman of Psychiatry*

University of California, Davis—DONALD G. LANGSLEY, *chairman of psychiatry*

University of Connecticut (Hartford)—RONALD M. WINTROB, *associate professor of psychiatry*

Drew Postgraduate Medical School (Los Angeles)—J. ALFRED CANNON, *chairman of psychiatry*

University of South Florida (Tampa)—WALTER AFIELD, *chairman of psychiatry*

University of Hawaii (Honolulu)—JOHN F. MCDERMOTT, JR., *chairman of psychiatry*

Southern Illinois University (Springfield)—WILLIAM L. STEWART, *professor and chairman, Department of Family Practice*

Louisiana State University at Shreveport—CHARLES S. SCHOBER, *head of psychiatry*

Mayo Clinic (Rochester, Minn.)—RICHARD M. STEINHILBER, *chairman of psychiatry*

Michigan State University (East Lansing)—ALLEN J. ENELOW, *chairman of psychiatry*

University of Minnesota at Duluth—ROBERT E. CARTER, *dean*

University of Missouri at Kansas City—CHARLES B. WILKINSON, *assistant dean of curriculum*

Mt. Sinai Hospital (New York City)—EDWARD JOSEPH, *professor of psychiatry*

University of Nevada (Reno)—DEWITT C. BALDWIN, JR., *director, Division of Behavioral Sciences*

State University of New York at Stony Brook—STANLEY F. YOLLES, *chairman of psychiatry*

Medical College of Ohio at Toledo—MARVIN GOTTLIEB, *department of psychiatry*

Rush Medical College (Chicago)—ALFRED SOLOMON, *acting chairman of psychiatry*

University of Texas at Houston—LOUIS A. FAILLACE, *director, Program in Psychiatry*

University of Texas at Lubbock—DAN CROY, *assistant dean for student affairs*

University of Texas at San Antonio—ROBERT L. LEON, *chairman of psychiatry*

Eastern Virginia (Norfolk)—RICHARD E. DAVIS, *associate dean, School of Medicine*

New Chairmen in Established Schools

Dartmouth College (Hanover, N.H.)—PETER WHYBROW, *chairman of psychiatry*

University of Kentucky (Lexington)—ARNOLD LUDWIG, *chairman of psychiatry*

State University of New York at Albany—ALAN M. KRAFT, *chairman of psychiatry*

University of Vermont (Burlington)—F. PATRICK McKEGNEY, *chairman of psychiatry*

Residents and Students

University of California at Davis—JON MANDELBAUM, *medical student*

University of Hawaii (Honolulu)—RON KWON, *medical student*

Michigan State University (East Lansing)—ALAN BARNES, *resident*

Stanford University (Stanford, Calif.)—SAM BENSON, *resident*

Resource Consultants

ALEX ADSETT, *professor of psychiatry, McMaster University, Hamilton, Ontario, Canada*

BERNARD BANDLER, *chief, Division of Manpower and Training, National Institute of Mental Health*

WALTER E. BARTON, *medical director, American Psychiatric Association*

F. PATRICK OKURA, *special assistant to the director, National Institute of Mental Health*

WILLIAM E. BUNNEY, *acting director, Division of Narcotic Addiction and Drug Abuse, National Institute of Mental Health*

HILLIARD JASON, *director, Office of Medical Education Research and Development, Michigan State University*

HARVEY L. P. RESNIK, *director, Center for Studies of Suicide Prevention, National Institute of Mental Health*

JOHN ROMANO, *Distinguished University Professor of Psychiatry, University of Rochester School of Medicine*

WALTER W. SHERVINGTON, *chief, Psychiatry Training Branch, National Institute of Mental Health*

ROBERT L. STUBBLEFIELD, *president, American Association of Chairmen of Departments of Psychiatry (AACDP)*

BRYCE TEMPLETON, *National Board of Medical Examiners*

CLAUDEWELL S. THOMAS, *director, Division of Mental Health Service Programs, National Institute of Mental Health*

THOMAS WEBSTER, *chief, Continuing Education Branch, Division of Manpower and Training, National Institute of Mental Health*

VAN BUREN O. HAMMETT, *professor and chairman, Department of Psychiatry, Hahnemann Medical College*

Conference Secretary: JOAN L. HOWARD

Mental Health Education
in the
New Medical Schools

⋟⋟⋟⋟⋟⋟⋟⋟ Part One ⋞⋞⋞⋞⋞⋞⋞⋞

Undergraduate Psychiatric Education

⋟⋟⋟⋟⋟⋟⋟⋟⋟⋟⋟⋟⋟⋞⋞⋞⋞⋞⋞⋞⋞⋞⋞⋞

As we enter the second third of the decade of the seventies, it has become apparent that medical education in general and psychiatric education in particular are undergoing remarkable changes. The title of this book reflects one of the most important changes: that psychiatry is beginning to see its role as one of the mental health professions, working with others already in the field. At the same time the once secure role of the psychiatry department (which was secure for such a brief span, less than thirty years) is being challenged from two sources. First is a trend toward interdisciplinary teaching in place of the more traditional department-controlled blocks of teaching time. The other challenge comes from the basic science side. After a difficult struggle to get preclinical time for behavioral science assigned to departments of psychiatry, the emergence of the concept of departments of behavioral science threatens to take this achievement away from the psychiatrists. Many psychiatrist-scientists, unlike their clinician colleagues, believe that this is the most interesting and exciting part of psychiatric education.

In the first two chapters, these new developments are described and the case is argued for both. Dr. Adsett describes a unique matrix management model for creating a multidisciplinary

1

medical education program in which psychiatry, like every other department, has no control over undergraduate medical education time or content. The input of psychiatry is into multidisciplinary planning committees. This development is not entirely new, and teaching by committee in a multidisciplinary format has been done before. But it is receiving increasing attention today and Adsett's description of the McMaster University model is particularly timely. Dr. Resnik argues in his chapter that the clinicians should teach clinical science and that basic behavioral science deserves a department of its own. This proposal is being debated, sometimes with great heat, at many medical schools and other training institutions. In the conference discussion that followed, summarized in Chapter Three, the greatest degree of division occurred around the issue of the separate behavioral science department.

Undergraduate Programs:
The McMaster Experience

C. A. ADSETT

*L*earning to become a physician is a complex business. To describe some of the varied issues involved I first give a brief orientation to the new medical school program at McMaster University and then discuss medical education in general, focusing on the achievement of integration and flexibility in undergraduate programs. Finally, I address some specific issues relevant to psychiatry: goals of psychiatric education for medical students and various methods of achieving these goals.

McMaster Medical School

McMaster is a small university with seven thousand students located in Hamilton, Ontario—a metropolitan area of four hundred thousand people, located on the southwest edge of Lake Ontario. The new medical school opened its doors in September 1969, admitting a class of twenty students; and only three years later the freshman class had sixty-four students. A distinguishing feature of the McMaster Medical School is that from the beginning there was a conscious philosophy on the part of the dean and his senior colleagues to emphasize integrated programs rather than powerful departmental empires. Interdependence and cooperation were given higher value than independence and competition, so that an almost communal environment has emerged. The integrated undergraduate education program extends for three years on an eleven-month basis and is divided into four phases, several horizontal programs, and some electives.

Phase I lasts ten weeks and is intended to help the student move from a traditional didactic educational system to a small group tutorial system which focuses on self-learning and problem-solving. While the major emphasis in this phase is on the process of learning, there is also considerable content providing an overview of the structure and function of the body and exploring physical and psychosocial aspects of growth and development. Phase II extends ten weeks and presents the human organism's response to stimuli at all levels, including cells, tissues, whole body, and behavior. During this phase the student is introduced to the content of microbiology, immunology, general pathology, and psychopathology through exploring in some depth a series of clinical models. These models include bioenergetics, streptococcal infection, neoplasia, ischaemia, and psychological depression. In Phase III the student explores the various body systems for a forty-week period. The systems are divided into five units: hemopoetic gastrointestinal; cardiorespiratory; nervous locomotor; endocrine reproduction; and kidney and body fluids. During this period the student learns basic mechanisms of pathophysiology and is introduced to clinical skills of medical history-taking and physical diagnosis.

The horizontal programs, extending throughout Phases I, II, and III, provide a series of experiences which emphasize attitudes and various clinical management skills. These experiences are not readily integrated into the so-called vertical aspects of the program but linkages are established wherever possible. Horizontal programs include a supervised interviewing experience in Phases I and II and a supervised clinical team experience in Phase III. The student has an opportunity to work with a community physician in Phase II and Phase III. Throughout the three phases, aspects of health care delivery are discussed with the students. A series of seminars consider such topics as death and dying and ethics and legal aspects related to medicine. A four-week elective after Phase II and a six-week elective after Phase III are left completely open for the student to decide on the use of his time in consultation with his student advisor.

Phase IV is a forty-eight–week clinical clerkship experience which includes sixteen weeks of elective time. Because of difficulties in providing an integrated learning experience during the clinical clerkship, I will go into it in more detail later.

Achieving Integration

Administrative Organization. To set up an integrated educational system, the faculty selected an M. D. Education Committee of about ten faculty of varying disciplines who showed qualities of imagination, flexibility, and willingness to approach problems from various angles and work together. This group continually reinforces student needs for a forward-looking general medical education consonant with the overall goals of the medical school, rather than emphasizing individual faculty or departmental needs or interests. Individuals on the education committee are given charge of different phases of the educational program and each phase is steered by a multidisciplinary planning group responsible to the education committee through the particular phase chairman. Each phase, in turn, is broken down into units with multidisciplinary unit-planning committees which are kept small in order to be effective working groups. Students are represented on all these committees and encouraged to function as creative individuals working toward common goals rather than lobbying for student power. We found that if these multidisciplinary committees become too large they are ineffective, or if one strong person tends to dominate the group the biases of this individual could result in an imbalance in the educational program.

The functional organization of this integrated educational system was borrowed from the matrix management model, a grid model with the departmental lines running vertically and the program lines running horizontally. The program director and his co-workers—in this case, the education committee—are responsible for carrying out the educational program but rely on support from and interaction with the various departments and department chairmen to obtain personnel resources. This model removes some power of the department chairman and puts a great deal of the action into programs. The chairman is responsible for maintaining the professional growth of his faculty in their specific disciplines and for specific department activities as well as providing resources for interdepartmental programs.

While the matrix management model for educational programs has an exciting potential, it is not without its problems. Anxiety levels are high when faculty are taken out of the secure niche of their department and have to integrate their teaching activities into a broad multidisciplinary program. Moreover, power struggles can develop between department chairmen and program directors unless the system is set up to allow good communication to and from the faculty administration. At McMaster, communication takes place through the chairman of the education committee reporting to the faculty executive and the faculty council, both of which bodies include the department chairmen.

Educational Objectives. A primary task of the planning groups is to create clear statements of learning objectives, in a general way for the overall program by the education committee and in increasingly specific form by the phase and unit-planning committees. At the unit level these learning objectives are presented to the students in the form of identified key questions and problems for the students to probe, study, and try to resolve. In this way, we emphasize learning and problem-solving and avoid the pitfalls of an encyclopedic approach to content. This selection of objectives and formulation into broad clinical problems, if it is truly multidisciplinary, is an extremely difficult process requiring a great deal of attention by the planning committees and a high degree of group judgment. Once these fairly specific learning objectives are developed, a variety of learning resources including audiovisual media are prepared and the students' learning schedule is flexibly designed to allow them to explore the learning resources with considerable freedom as to their own time and pace.

Starting from a real-life clinical problem of dramatic interest the student is stimulated to explore different parameters of the problem. Using an array of learning resources the student gains an understanding of many of the basic mechanisms of disordered functions. This format provides a comprehensive and exciting learning experience for the student as long as he does not get so carried away with interesting clinical details that he neglects the essential exercise of exploring the basic concepts necessary to truly understand the problem. The following is an example of a problem presented to students in the nervous system unit in Phase III:

A fifty-three-year-old male schoolteacher is directed to a physician by the school principal, who describes him as increasingly neglectful of his appearance and functioning poorly at work for several weeks. The patient complains of being slowed down and tired, yet has difficulty sleeping at night. He lives alone since his wife was killed in an auto accident two years earlier and his two children live in distant cities. The physician notes the patient is circumstantial, forgetful, apathetic, and possibly depressed. Physical examination is normal except for slight hypertension of 145/95. (Students are shown a real or simulated patient.)

Some questions which could be explored by the tutorial group: (1) How could you go about testing this man's mental status? (2) Given data from his performance on the Wechsler Adult Intelligence scale, which subtests would interest you most and why? (3) To what extent could these symptoms be due to depression? (4) If depression is a likely diagnosis, what is the likelihood of suicide? How would you explore this? (5) What is the relationship between sleep disturbance and depression? (6) Could this man's symptoms be due to an organic process in spite of lack of neurological findings on physical examination? (7) What kinds of medical and radiological tests would be most valuable in assessing organic damage and what findings might be present? (8) If dementia were to develop, what might be the pathological process? (9) What social, interpersonal, or family factors might be relevant to this man's problem? What community resources might be helpful in managing this situation? (10) If the man improved on antidepressant medication, what would be a possible biochemical explanation for his symptoms and their improvement?

Resource People: *Dr. S. Smith and Dr. J. Cleghorn.* Resources: *(1) Videotape on "Examples of Psychopathology"; (2) Videotape on "Psychological Testing"; (3) Slide Tape—Depression Model; (4) Freedman and Kaplan,* Comprehensive Textbook of Psychiatry; *(5) Holmes,* Introduction to Clinical Neurology, *pages 177–178; (6) Meyer and Gross,* Clinical Psychiatry, *3rd Edition, Slater and Roth, pages 610–629; (7) Shepherd, Lader, and Rodnight,* Clinical Pharmacology, *pages 214–224; (8)* Drug Treatment in Psychiatry, *Veterans Administration, January 1970, pages 17–24.*

The student is thus directed into biological, psychological, and social areas of learning in order to understand and manage this problem. The integration of basic sciences with clinical medicine has not been a serious problem at McMaster, where basic scientists work in clinical departments rather than in separate basic science departments. The integration of knowledge from different disciplines, however, has been much more difficult, because our faculty have trained as narrow specialists. Psychiatry particularly has problems, for while medical disciplines are developing into highly sophisticated technological sciences, social psychiatry (distinct from biological psychiatry) is becoming a complex managerial science residing on the fringe of medicine. Biologically oriented physicians and social psychiatrists find it difficult to talk and to share teaching seminars and research projects and to care for patients together in clinical settings. Because clinical behavioral science is less advanced as a systematic body of knowledge than most of the other medical sciences, it has difficulty competing with them when presented purely in an academic theoretical form.

In our experience, behavioral sciences are best demonstrated in relationship to real patient problems. Teaching sessions with patients who have well-defined behavioral problems and where a psychiatrist is in attendance have usually been productive. One multidisciplinary learning session in the cardiovascular unit used the format of a patient who had become delirious after cardiac surgery. A cardiac surgeon, an intensive care nurse, and a psychiatrist explored with the students the basis and management of this problem. The students came away with the message that this is not just a biological or behavioral problem but a complex situation involving interaction among a variety of influences and requiring assessment of different kinds of data.

Lack of Integration. It is vital when setting up a multidisciplinary educational program to discriminate between areas of medical practice and education whose lack of integration is due to political organization or chauvinistic attitudes and those areas which lack integration because no real relationship between the disciplines or topics exists. For example, in our growth and development program some areas of physical and psychosocial development, such as learning disabilities in young children or adolescent problems, where integration seemed highly desirable were sometimes dealt with separately because the pediatrician and the psychiatrist each wanted to do his own thing. On the other hand, in the field of psychiatry, for example, the gap between molecular biology or basic neurosciences and clinical behavior is in many cases so vast that any attempt to integrate them at this stage of our knowledge appeared artificial and contrived and merely made the learning experience for the student more difficult.

Faculty Roles. In addition to being planners, faculty also serve as resource people, tutors, and student advisors, so that a psychiatrist might be called upon to play any one or more of these four roles. The resource faculty member is an expert in a circumscribed area of knowledge, and his task is to prepare learning resources to meet educational objectives applicable to that area and to function as a leader in seminar discussions, demonstrations, or patient-oriented teaching sessions. As this is a fairly traditional role with the person functioning in his own area of expertise he is usually quite comfortable.

Since the students' learning is focused around a small group tutorial, the tutor is a key person as he guides a small group of four to eight students through a ten-week segment of the course. The general tutor concentrates on the learning process of his students, rather than on content, and serves to stimulate and guide his students to learn how to formulate questions, use learning resources, analyze data, and discuss their ideas with the rest of the group. The tutor is the faculty person who helps the student integrate his knowledge as well as the one who works with the student to evaluate his progress, so he is in a key position to influence the student toward a comprehensive approach to problems. He is also in a role which is new and extremely difficult for him. We grossly underestimated the lack of skill and experience of our faculty to perform this integrating role, and during the past two years we have expended as much time and energy educating faculty as we have in educating medical students. Currently tutor training is introducing faculty to small group dynamics and the problem-solving approach to learning. The trainee attends workshops and gains experience as an assistant tutor before becoming a tutor.

Psychiatrists usually have a comprehensive viewpoint and a knowledge of group dynamics but are often reluctant to function as tutors because they feel inadequate in helping the student with biological aspects of medicine. They are much more at home with the role of student advisor. As a student advisor, the faculty person periodically meets with his student during his three years at medical school to help him with his career plans, choice of electives, and any personal concerns.

Summary. At McMaster we possibly went overboard with integration in attempting to do too much too fast. Currently, our thinking is that partial integration seems both feasible and desirable with recognition of the fact that some areas cannot be integrated, at least given the current state of our knowledge. We also realize that students need to do some integrating themselves and can do so if presented with faculty who demonstrate attitudes of thinking and working in a multidisciplinary fashion.

Our experience suggests that the way to achieve an integrated educational program is through a multidisciplinary administrative system based on the matrix management model, through formulating educational objectives as clinical problems rather than attempting to integrate abstract theory, and finally through providing a variety of educational roles for all faculty to share, with special emphasis on the tutor role. Integration is achieved only at a high price in time and energy of faculty and financial cost. The logistics of an integrated program, including training faculty and achieving satisfactory communication among them, is exceedingly complex. Though I think partial integration in medical education is practical for a new medical school, I question whether it is either feasible or worth the effort for an established traditional school. On the other hand, where integration is achieved its influence spreads beyond education to produce productive changes in clinical and research activity patterns as well. At McMaster, educational integration has influenced the development of a committee and director of clinical programs which is a multidisciplinary group overseeing and coordinating clinical programs within the Health Sciences Centre. Coordination in research planning has developed with the formation of the Committee on Scientific Development, made up of researchers from various departments who do long-range planning and advise the faculty about resources required to achieve our research goals.

Achieving Flexibility

Variable Depth in Tutorial System. The trend in medical education in recent years is toward a program of variable length with the individuals' achievement of objectives determining the rate of progression. We have taken a different route at McMaster by opting for a fixed three-year program that achieves flexibility through variable depth. A completely individualized course would be out of the question in our situation, where the learning process is based on the group tutorial which capitalizes on the emotional and academic learning derived from interaction with a heterogeneous group of peers. We hope our students will be better prepared as a result of their tutorial experience to work in settings where teamwork is vitally important. Physicians are too often prima donnas, much better adapted for solo work than working with closely interacting groups, and it is likely that the traditional impersonal programs or the completely individualized programs contribute to this phenomenon. The tutorial system requires students to cover the same topic in a unit of time, but otherwise the student is free to learn in his own way and at his own pace, and there is great variability in the depth, and to a lesser extent the breadth, with which individual students explore different parameters of problems. A particular problem might stimulate one student to go deeply into the behavioral area; another student to emphasize physiology; while a third student might spend more time on the pathology. However, all students are expected to attain the basic objectives for the unit. For example, in Phase I students studying the problem of pain would all be expected to know some basic anatomy and function of the nervous system such that they could outline the mechanism of pain in a specific situation. They would also be expected to know that psychosocial factors can influence the experiencing and presentation of pain and that indeed pain can exist in some situations as a purely psychological mechanism without a body lesion.

Our experience has led us to be impressed with the group tutorial, both as a format for critical learning and as a source of group support to students during a stressful period of their lives. As our tutors increase their skills they are also becoming much more comfortable with the tutorial as a medium for evaluation. It not only allows the student to evaluate himself but gives him the benefit of evaluation by a faculty person who has worked closely with him and knows him fairly well after a ten-week period, as well as evaluation by several of his peers who have also interacted closely with him for ten weeks. It should be mentioned that tutors are not restricted to relating to students in group tutorials and at times see students individually.

Electives. The introduction of electives has brought more flexibility and excitement to both students and faculty. Electives stimulate the student and allow him a change of pace and to explore an area of his own interest. They also allow the student having difficulty a chance to catch up.

Electives have dangers, however. The marked tracking in some medical schools in the United States, where students concentrate very early and almost exclusively on topics related to a particular career choice, seems to me a dangerous trend. I believe our graduates need a broad medical doctor degree which enables them to obtain a license to practice medicine without restriction, and yet students are often trained to a competent level in only a narrow area. Many, if not most, medical students do not know what they want at an early phase of their education. I have seen students fix on a career at an early stage because they were encouraged to do so and, as a result, close their minds to learning in many broad areas of medicine. Moreover, some of these students later discover that they have made an inappropriate career choice and need to recycle their education. Such tracking requires a superb student advisor system in which the student advisor knows the student extremely well, and I have yet to see such a system in a medical school.

If we look at medical education as a continuum consisting of various periods with goals in each, Period I might be considered the preparatory or premedical university stage. Here, hopefully, students obtain a broad general education including some science and arts as well as skills in self-learning, problem-solving, and increasing personal maturity. Period II or medical school proper, as far as McMaster is concerned, provides a comprehensive basic medical education which graduates a general physician prepared to go on learning in specialized tracks of his own choosing. The third period, that of residency training, can be looked at as a clinical apprenticeship along one of three tracks: medical science; clinical specialty (primary care or consulting); or family practice. Since a rotating internship is fast becoming extinct, the graduate physician usually begins his residency track immediately upon graduation. In Canada we are becoming aware of the general public's concern about the superspecialization within medicine—witness the many jokes, such as the one about the physician who deals only with the left ear. The public is demanding that areas with great need such as primary care be adequately serviced. It may not be too many years hence that the medical student will not have a completely free choice of career specialty.

Summary. At McMaster, we have satisfied ourselves that a three-year program based on an eleven-month year is a satisfactory arrangement for both students and faculty and produces a student who meets our standard of competence. We have not attempted to completely individualize our educational program, preferring to retain the fixed time period and develop flexibility through variation in depth along different parameters of the students' learning. We focus on the small group tutorial as a way of building support, heterogeneity of interest, and personal interaction in medical education. We are impressed with the value of electives and have seen some of the most exciting learning experiences for students come from electives they have designed themselves. However, we are also concerned about the dangers of carrying electives to an extreme with resulting fragmentation of the student's education at an early point in his development.

Goals of Undergraduate Psychiatric Education

Psychiatry's role in undergraduate education is not to seduce students into the specialty of psychiatry but to improve their functioning as physicians of whatever specialty. More specifically, our goals include: awareness of the psychosocial aspects of behavior which relates to problems presented by patients; awareness of the subtleties of patient-physician interaction; awareness of the ecological context from whence patients come; awareness of various paradigms related to understanding behavior, including biological, social, and psychological models.

An integrated curriculum such as the one I discussed earlier provides a logical format for making psychiatry relevant to what a physician does. Human behavior may be taught for many hours in a separate psychiatry course, yet if this learning is not reinforced in other parts of the educational program it often has little impact on the overall functioning of the student.

A continuing experience with patients from the first week of medical school provides the student with an opportunity to learn the fundamentals of the complex art of interviewing, including observational skills and awareness of doctor-patient interaction. Learning about human behavior, more than any other learning that goes on in medical school, must personally involve the student so that feelings are tied in with theoretical learning. The student should be closely supervised when he is exposed to the emotional impact of working with patients, as learning cannot take place if the student is overwhelmed by his own anxiety.

Not only does the student need to learn to observe behavioral data, but he requires an easily understood framework on which to fit the myriad bits of information in a meaningful way. Students are introduced to a variety of paradigms one at a time, giving them a chance to see examples of its use before moving to another model. Our teaching experience suggests that the sequence in this learning is very important. Students can learn and accept broad, simple models more readily at first than they can specific, complex types.

For example, we start with broad scientific concepts: the adaptation model provides a framework for viewing health and disease; systems theory helps students appreciate that what is happening in the family and in the community has a bearing on the individual problem. Social paradigms, such as role theory, aid the student in examining family and work relationships and help him understand how role conflicts may arise. The first psychological model students encounter is learning theory because it is readily demonstrable and the student has no difficulty understanding how a variety of behaviors are developed through reinforcement from the environment. The interviewing experience introduces the transactional model as it focuses on behavior between people which students actually observe. After they have become familiar with transactional concepts and developed skill in observing these in real-life situations, students are much more likely to be ready to look at psychodynamic and psychoanalytic models without tremendous resistance. Because psychodynamic models have complex theory and much of their behavioral data is inferred, rather than directly observed, students either get lost or turned off by them if they are presented too early.

Alliance of Psychiatry with Family Medicine

McMaster Medical School to a large extent uses traditional clinical facilities which existed before it opened. As a result, our nondepartmental philosophy has not been implemented as much in the clinical clerkship as it has in the first three phases. Our faculty is now developing a variety of multidisciplinary clinical settings for training students. These settings exist on three levels: level one is primary care, which includes a family health care centre operated by teams of family physicians with nurse practitioners and using specialists as consultants. A second primary care model involves a mixture of specialists and general practitioners who provide either episodic or continuing care. A third model is an emergency service which provides prompt emergency treatment with follow-up. At Level Two, which we call special ambulatory care, the various specialty clinics manage more complex medical problems, and provide consultation and education for primary care physicians. Level Three, in-patient care, is divided into two types of units: the undifferentiated unit, which is a multidisciplinary type of ward, and a differentiated unit which is a highly specialized unit requiring specalized equipment and specially trained staff.

We are currently modifying our clinical clerkship from department-oriented, hospital-based training so that half the students' clinical experience is in a comprehensive primary care setting. From this area the student can then follow selected patients into the various areas of both ambulatory and in-patient specialty medicine, where he can work as a peripheral member of the specialty team. To evolve the clinical clerkship into a broad, community-oriented experience, the first step was to combine two department programs which have major common areas of interest. Internal medicine and surgery have combined their approach to medical-surgical problems; pediatrics and obstetrics have a joint approach to clinical aspects of reproduction and growth and development; and the marriage of family medicine and psychiatry provides an integrated eight-week experience in a primary care clinical setting with strong psychiatric input.

This combination of family medicine and psychiatry seems logical for several reasons. McMaster, recognizing the need for front-line physicians who can handle the large volume of ambulatory care, is committed to producing more primary care physicians and upgrading the training of the family physician to better play a key role in the health care system. Because such physicians will be called upon to provide comprehensive, remedial, and preventive care it is imperative that they know a great deal about the psychosocial aspects of clinical medicine. The family physician's interest in the whole family as a social unit through which to deliver health care is reflected in our department of psychiatry's strong orientation toward examining the family unit and providing family therapy, rather than looking exclusively at the individual. Our psychiatry department also has great interest in preventing various social problems in the community which lead to maladaptive behavior. As psychiatrists, we are well aware that we will never have the resources to cope with the vast number of psychosocial problems in the community. Hence, we welcome the opportunity to be resource people to the primary care physician, who can be our arms and legs in grappling with these problems on a broad front. This cooperative relationship is particularly effective in the area of preventive psychiatry, where the family physician can do a great deal to help parents and families with their growing children. Such individuals rarely get to psychiatrists until the late stages of psychopathology in adolescence or adulthood. Although I have concentrated here on the relationship of psychiatrists and family physicians, our department does a great deal of teaching as well with various health-related professions in an attempt to improve their handling of behavioral problems at the primary care level.

During the psychiatry–family medicine rotation the clinical clerk is assigned to a primary health care team consisting of a family physician, a nurse practitioner, and various resource people, including a psychiatrist and social worker. The student assumes responsibility for the health care of many families under close supervision of the team. In addition, each student carries out family therapy with a couple of families under supervision of a psychiatrist. Much of the academic input comes from specific seminars in clinical psychiatry, as well as joint teaching seminars in which both family physicians and psychiatrists take part. The student also has opportunities for specific learning in psychiatry outside the primary care setting, such as learning from patients who were referred from the primary care unit to a differentiated psychiatric unit or taking calls at a crisis intervention center to gain experience with acute psychological crises. Finally, visits to a large mental hospital enable the student to see problems he is unlikely to encounter during his eight weeks in a primary care setting.

To summarize, our clinical clerkship is evolving into a broad, interdisciplinary experience with more emphasis on ambulatory care. Our integrated clinical model uses the primary care physician (family physician, general internist, or general pediatrician) as a key person in the health care system with strong support from many specialists. This model is analogous to our educational model where the tutor plays a key role supported by a variety of expert resource faculty.

As departmental barriers are removed, psychiatry and family medicine have been drawn together, because the aim of psychiatry is to teach medical students how to be better physicians. Further, psychiatry and family medicine have many common interests and much to learn from each other. It is possible that psychiatry may play a more useful role in solving our enormous health problems than it has in the past as it finds a viable role within the medical profession providing resource people and educators to the primary care deliverers.

Behavioral Sciences: Wherefrom, Whether, and W(h)ither?

H. L. P. RESNIK

≈≈≈≈≈≈≈≈≈≈≈≈≈≈≈⋘⋘⋘⋘⋘⋘⋘⋘⋘⋘

*W*hen you don't know where you are going, any road will take you there; so it has seemed with the behavioral sciences. I do not propose to identify all those names and combinations of names variously grouped under the behavioral sciences.* The Group for the Advancement of Psychiatry, in their report (1962) on the preclinical teaching of psychiatrists, called the behavioral sciences the integrated study of the biological, psychological, and sociocultural facets of human behavior. Many would similarly describe psychiatry.

Obviously, one needs to agree on the behavioral sciences in order to objectify what they are expected to do. The important fall-out from such efforts at definition is to force departments of psychiatry to look at their own reasons for existence. Nurnberger (1969) felt strongly that the biological bases of behavior were neglected in

---

* I appreciate very much the exchange of ideas on this subject with F. Marian Bishop, Ph.D., and Elmer F. Bertsch, M.A.

behavioral science teaching in the medical schools and presented a brief for behavioral genetics, hormonal chemistry, functional neuro-anatomy, and behavioral neuropsychology. The biological bases are the subject matter of psychiatry. In the 1969 report of the National Academy of Sciences and the Social Science Research Council, nine behavioral and social sciences (they were not sep-arated) are identified—and in their interpretation psychiatry itself becomes one of but different from the others. How that important decision came about is unclear. The others were anthropology, economics, geography, history, linguistics, political science, psy-chology, and sociology. Each of these was the subject of a special committee report. That on psychiatry, edited by Hamburg (1969) and entitled *Psychiatry As a Behavioral Science,* was produced by six chairmen of psychiatry in major medical schools. At the time they were writing, I believe, their schools had neither a department of behavioral sciences nor any department titles which included the words *behavioral sciences.* Yet I know from personal experience, since I trained in one of these programs, that the behavioral sciences were indeed an important part of the resident's education. Were they saying that a properly conceptualized psychiatry department in fact is a behavioral science department as well?

I certainly cannot quarrel with that implication. Their mono-graph encompasses the breadth of psychiatry. Yet the title is some-what disquieting. Psychiatry as a behavioral science? Surely one must infer that psychiatry is the medical application of the science(s) of behavior. The monograph points to psychiatry's appropriate scien-tific position at the interface between the biological and behavioral sciences. I prefer to see the biologic and behavioral interfaces en-compassed by psychiatry. Perhaps this is an exercise in semantics, but anything that is at an interface is only a point of reference. Perhaps psychiatry is indeed only a transitional point on a con-tinuum of the behavioral sciences. History shows clearly that psychi-atrists (Adolf Meyer comes immediately to mind) have led the way in attempting to understand the individual as a biologic and psychologic entity operating within a social context unit. But I have difficulty considering psychiatry a behavioral science. I believe psychiatrists can be trained in and use behavioral techniques but when they use them they are not behavioral scientists, unless they have training in two doctoral fields. Of course, in that case they have "the best of all possible worlds" and can slide in and out of their medical credentials. The word *psychiatry* derives from the Greek roots *psyche* (the human mind) and *iatreia* (healing), which leads to *iatrikos* (pertaining to a physician). Thus, the early use of the word succeeded in distinguishing physicians who studied the mind from nonphysicians. In other words, even then, the word was "Will the real doctors stand up?" In the medical schools of only five to ten years ago, behavioral scientists could not.

Variables in Creating Departments

There are numerous precedents for the evolution of departments in medical schools. Departments of neurology were created from departments of medicine, from which pediatrics also separated. Departments of surgery have been even more prolific—spawning orthopedics, neurosurgery, and anesthesiology, among a number of separate departments. The medical study of the mind, or psychiatry, emerged directly from the perceived interrelationship between the nervous system and certain "nervous states." And, indeed, it has not been long—perhaps forty years—since the vast majority of psychiatrists practiced neurology as well. They performed this double duty in what first were called departments of neurology and then neurology and psychiatry. Ultimately, as psychiatry emerged in its own right, it received separate department status, although there are still vestiges of this antiquated relationship in departments called psychiatry and neurology. What a professor that chairman must be! Dr. Robert Felix' successful splitting off of NIMH from NIH was probably the most influential move in recognizing psychiatry as a science. Moreover, it also set in motion Dr. Stanley Yolles' leadership in recognizing the behavioral sciences. Like psychiatry's emergence, the gradual recognition of the behavioral sciences has been attended by resistance and nonacceptance (which in some areas continue today).

Straus (1965) answered in detail the "what" and "how" questions concerning the operation of the first administratively separate department of behavioral sciences in the United States. His goals were sixfold: (1) to present a historical and comparative-cul-

tures perspective as a basis for considering the impact of technological
and social change on the nature of contemporary and future medical
science and on forms of medical care; (2) to establish the essential
interdependence of social, psychological, environmental, and biological phenomena in determining the genesis, distribution, diagnosis,
course, and management of the general health needs of society and
of specific disease processes, as well as to examine the beliefs, attitudes, values, and activities associated with human response to illness
in general and to specific forms of illness; (3) to provide understanding of the processes of communication and human relationship
basic to the interaction of health personnel with patients and with
each other, the social structure of hospitals and other health organizations, and the impact of illness on the fulfillment of family, occupational, and community roles; (4) to elucidate the nature of
medicine as a complex system of human behavior, its relationship
to such other behavior systems as religion, government, and economics, and factors involved in the organization and distribution
of health resources in order to bring the benefits of modern medical
science to bear on the varying needs and health problems of different
segments of society, when and where they exist; (5) to introduce
statistical concepts and methods and an orientation to behavioral
science methodology as these are applied to medical inquiry and
understanding; and (6) to help students understand the various
modes which facilitate and impede communication and how to
apply communication skills to a variety of activities in the medical
setting.

　　What this definition does to the territoriality of a department
of psychiatry is obvious. It is threatened! Thus, the capability of
dealing with a number of issues and needs for which responsibility
had been scattered and often absent becomes centralized in a new
department, which also provides skilled professionals who can
handle questions the government and citizens are currently asking
about the organization and delivery of health care. Straus noted
prophetically that "to the extent that the behavioral sciences are
truly functional in helping the physician meet the many requirements which are associated with social and medical change, they
will become fully accepted as sciences basic to medicine." That
acceptance has indeed come to pass. The issue I want to consider

is, given that acceptance, what has been done and can be done to acknowledge it?

Straus observed that there were no distinct patterns for locating behavioral science activity in a school's table of organization or its curriculum. Almost every school has behavioral science teaching time in the curriculum. Increasingly, interdepartmental collaborations have resulted in more basic-science psychiatry, as some have called the behavioral sciences. This term is characteristic of psychiatrically oriented thinking, since it implies that the behavioral sciences cannot or do not stand alone.

As recently as ten years ago behavioral science teaching strength in medical schools was minimal (Von Mering, 1969; Webster, 1967; Zimet, 1969). Frequently, one literally had to search for a behavioral scientist consultant within the medical school. When located, he would probably be in a department of psychiatry, or a department of preventive (or community) medicine, or much more frequently now in a newly organized department of family medicine. Usually he could be identified in the catalog with the second-class designation of Instructor in Psychiatry (Sociology), or Assistant Professor of Preventive Medicine (Medical Sociology), or any of a variety of permutations that said implicitly: "You are not a physician but a second-class citizen." He rarely could vote in the faculty of medicine. Where a university contained a school of public health, there, most frequently, was the nucleus of behavioral science teaching strength, a strength infrequently called upon in the education of medical students. Furthermore, many medical centers were located far from the parent campus where course work in graduate programs in psychology, sociology, and anthropology were viewed as irrelevant to medical student education. I can recall my concern as a psychology and English major that I might not find a seat in a medical school. I remember the comments about the "lack of advanced biology, chemistry, or bacteriology courses in my records" that I heard at interviews. The truth of the matter may be that many of us psychiatrists were drawn from a pool of behavioral science undergraduate and graduate students. As we accepted the medical rites, we also influenced these rituals by our proneness to acknowledge and understand what our colleagues in sociology, anthropology, psychology, and humanism were teaching.

As late as 1967 Webster, while surveying psychiatry curriculum time, identified only two separate departments of behavioral sciences (Kentucky and Temple) and one called medical psychology (Oregon). He also referred to psychiatry and behavioral science as one and the same in the title of his paper, as well as in the text. He referred to instruction in the behavioral sciences as an increasingly significant part of preclinical curriculum. His report revealed the then prevalent curriculum concept of preclinical-clinical dichotomies which held that students needed grounding in basic sciences before being let loose on patients.

Administrative Creativity

The establishment of a division, section, or committee to highlight and shelter all those nonmedical aliens has taxed the administrative creativity of many chairmen and deans. Such recognition is not limited to departments of psychiatry. We are seeing the behavioral sciences increasingly recognized in departments of preventive medicine, community health, family medicine, and community medicine. And they are also appearing in schools of public health and allied health sciences, as well as schools of nursing, dentistry, and the ministry. Where the behavioral science group has become strong in the medical school (probably by dint of a charismatic leader) or where department leadership has become au courant, a departmental rechristening may take place. For example, in established medical schools we now have departments of psychiatry and behavioral sciences (Johns Hopkins and Oklahoma) and psychiatry and human behavior (Maryland, Michigan State). There are many more permutations in the new schools. The handwriting is clear—nonmedical contributions must be recognized. This process to me is academic binary fission in its earliest stages—when there is, as yet, an unequal separation of nuclear material. Recognition of the behavioral sciences appears as an appended afterthought.

A more or less equal separation can occur through evolution, as at USC where an incumbent chairman of psychiatry, Dr. Edward Stainbrook chose to head the newly created department of human behavior. Or the separation can be along traditional lines, such as separate departments of psychiatry and medical psychology (Oregon). The process can be slow, or it may spring full blown from the administrative brow—as it most commonly appears to do in the new medical schools. The Kentucky plan came from Dean William Willard's earlier decision to include behavioral scientists on his planning staff, and it predated an operating department of psychiatry. Dean George T. Harrell at Hershey went one better by establishing both a department of behavioral science and a department of humanities very early in the formative stages of that school. He simply reallocated Straus's six objectives to two new departments.

The variety of names chosen in the new schools clearly indicates the struggle to achieve an identity. Human resources, human behavior, behavior and human services, psychology and the sciences of society, behavioral biology, medical social sciences, social perspectives—what a mind-expanding experience in name coining!* I am reminded of Lewis Carroll's *Through the Looking Glass* when Humpty Dumpty tells Alice "When I use a word . . . it means just what I choose it to mean." These names give little information other than about the varied interchangeability of words. I suspect all these new entities purport to do the same things.

We have come far from the 1967 Conference on Psychiatry and Medical Education where Simmons and Brosin (1969) traced the emerging role of the behavioral sciences in the medical schools. They reported the assumption (certainly confirmed today) that "the contribution of the behavioral sciences to medical education is in no way limited to psychiatry but has relevance for many if not all of the medical specialties." They felt it "too early to formulate and recommend any one pattern as entirely unsuitable."

My feeling is that there can be little behavioral science taught effectively in the medical schools without being placed at some time in a clinical context. The justification for behavioral sciences in the medical school is that they will provide research and teaching on issues related to understanding the delivery of care to individuals and their communities. Pure behavioral science is properly a graduate study independent of medicine. One teaches communication theory in order to better understand a patient; one teaches interpersonal dynamics in the context of familial influences on sickness;

* I am indebted to F. Marian Bishop for sharing her list with me. I understand that an updated survey will soon be forthcoming from R. Fletcher.

one talks of primate laboratories in relation to maternal deprivation and a laboratory model for studying depression. When one teaches about the maldistribution and unavailability of health services, it is in the context of understanding malnutrition and lead poisoning. Such teaching can be equally effective whether it emanates from a discrete department of behavioral sciences or from a division within psychiatry or community medicine. Any administrative structure less defined than that is ineffective. It is administratively very difficult to handle power issues by creating a new department, which probably explains why new departments of behavioral sciences or new locations such as family medicine are present more in emerging schools than in established schools. The latter are prone to amend the names of existing departments of psychiatry. The important variable to me is whether there is a continuing identification of and commitment to the behavioral sciences in the medical school curriculum. That leadership rests with the dean and is embodied in the curriculum committee. I am familiar with several schools which have superb courses in the behavioral sciences that commence in the first year and are woven throughout the medical school experience. What they have in common is not the discreteness of a department of behavioral sciences—for they are not—but rather a commitment within the philosophy of that school, for the teaching is truly an interdepartmental collaborative effort.

However, a demeaning of the behavioral sciences is *least* likely to occur where separate departments of psychiatry and behavioral sciences have been established. The facts of coexistence, shared power, teaching time, research space, and budget, as well as territoriality issues, are more workable under such circumstances. The behavioral scientists have their own champion, their chairman, to deal with the chairman of psychiatry as a peer. If I had to cite the most important elements in the success of behavioral science teaching programs, they would be the personalities of the chairman of psychiatry, the leader of behavioral science teaching, and the dean. The structure within the school, although important, is secondary. Excellent programs do exist in several models but they ride on the entente between the key administrators.

Around what issues differences occur is an ongoing discussion in many schools. Should responsibilities be delineated on clinical versus nonclinical assignments, basic versus applied research, or biophysical versus sociopsychologic investigations? I cannot begin to anticipate all the issues. What I have tried to say is that the questions of "wherefrom" and "whether" are more easily settled than that of "whither." My position is that the answer to "whither" for the behavioral sciences lies in a newly created department of behavioral science (or what you will call it) with a total involvement in the medical school that transcends traditional department lines. I see members of the behavioral sciences faculty organized around systems or programs into which they have a valued and clear input throughout the entire health science complex and not solely in the medical school. Responsibility for a beginning course in human behavior would rest with behavioral science, with the cooperation of related departments.

I suspect that I was invited to tackle this subject because of my involvement in a field—suicide prevention—that values and encourages contributions from all the behavioral sciences. To organize suicide prevention services requires clinicians to work closely with colleagues from other disciplines, primarily the behavioral sciences, and we feel we have collaborated successfully. In fact, I believe general psychiatry can be taught by starting medical students or residents in shared interprofessional training experiences originating in crisis intervention. In one month the gamut of psychiatric problems will be encountered, roles will be defined, and required learning experiences will become clear. And as students see what they will have to know—as it is defined for them by callers and colleagues—they will be hooked and motivated to learn relevant information.

Influences on Decision-Making

I conclude with some variables that I believe influence the establishment of departments of behavioral sciences in new schools and the separation of behavioral sciences from psychiatry in established schools. The four groupings are meant to be neither exhaustive nor exclusive nor insulting.

*White Knight Phenomenon.** The White Knight in *Alice*

* I first heard this described by Edmund Pellegrino.

in Wonderland was prepared to meet every contingency, to overcome every conceivable obstacle. However, in order to do so, he was so laden with paraphernalia that he could do nothing. Departments of psychiatry have, like the White Knight, grown and altered themselves to take up every new challenge. As problems grow larger new divisions are created to deal with them, such as forensic psychiatry, child psychiatry, adolescent psychiatry, community psychiatry, and behavioral sciences.

Four Furies. Budget, faculty slots, curriculum teaching time, and space are the four furies who shriek at every dean through the mouths of their chairmen. They add up to *power,* and few chairmen of psychiatry are willing to give up any of these to allow a dean to create a new department. One influence on budget and faculty slots is the lingering debate about whether behavioral scientists generate income against which a department can be operated. Questions of limited practice, offset income, and third-party payments are sore points with psychiatry faculty who deliver patient care. They see behavioral scientists as not pulling their fair share.

Walter Mitty Syndrome. The delivery of health care outside the medical centers is a national concern. Most psychiatrists have been poorly trained in epidemiology, sociology, anthropology, and economics. Psychiatrists must recognize that men trained in these fields have independent and useful contributions to make. The psychiatrist, by virtue of his M.D., cannot be the star of every performance. Where behavioral science has been located within a department of psychiatry, it has frequently served as handmaiden to the star.

Kekule Experience. An increasing number of deans must in their dreams synthesize new designs for medical school organization as well as curricular change. They must be willing to experiment with new models. A properly conceived and functioning department of behavioral sciences will appreciably lighten a dean's burden, as within it will often reside someone capable of helping his write his federal grant applications.

Psychiatry has grown like Topsy in response to many pressures, both medical and social. It is high time to recognize other expertise and redefine a new role for ourselves. Until that can be agreed upon—what it is we teach—we will be unable to evaluate the products of our training. If that agreement is reached, some departments of psychiatry may well spin off community psychiatry to behavioral sciences, child psychiatry to pediatrics, and forensic psychiatry to criminology. Then psychiatry will once again embrace the medical model from which it came and rejoin forces with internal medicine, family medicine, and Neurology as a clinical specialty. The "w(h)ither," then, is a combination of the *withering* of traditional psychiatry and the *whethering* of behavioral science as a discrete entity in the medical school.

᚜᚜᚜᚜᚜᚜᚜᚜᚜᚜᚜᚜᚜᚜᚜᚜᚜᚜᚜᚜᚜᚜᚜᚜᚜᚜᚜

Discussion

᚜᚜᚜᚜᚜᚜᚜᚜᚜᚜᚜᚜᚜᚜᚜᚜᚜᚜᚜᚜᚜᚜᚜᚜᚜᚜᚜

*T*he discussion of the McMaster experience began with Adsett's resummary of the matrix management model. He emphasized its characteristics as an alternative to departmental organization and pointed out that in this model much power and influence is taken away from the department and given to the members and director of the integrated multidisciplinary programs. The department chairman's responsibility becomes the career development of the people in his department plus those specific things that apply only to that discipline or field. This change not only removes some traditional powers of the chairman but does away with the customary battle for territory. There is no department of behavioral sciences at McMaster, but sociologists, social workers, psychologists, and other social scientists are in all departments, including the department of psychiatry. They can play a number of different roles in undergraduate education, including curriculum planners in a multidisciplinary group; tutors to help students with problem-solving and learning, working in small groups; and resource people for certain study programs. An example of the latter is a social anthropologist used to bring a cross-cultural perspective to the study of depression. Still another role is that of student advisor.

A question was raised about the emphasis on small group teaching in the McMaster model. Is it important to learn from close relationships with individual instructors, or does one pay a heavy price for the reduction of one-to-one contact of faculty with students? A related problem concerned those medical schools which have attempted some interdisciplinary teaching, particularly in behavioral science, but did not organize the entire medical school in the interdisciplinary, matrix-management style of McMaster University. Generally such attempts to do some, but not all, training this way have been less successful than those reported at McMaster.

An alternative approach to interdisciplinary teaching taken by the University of Nevada–Reno was described. At this school, multidisciplinary, nondepartmental teaching is begun at the undergraduate level, where health majors all take their courses together. There are three major divisions—biomedical, clinical, and behavioral. Some seven hundred students have declared majors in the health field, including medical technology, nursing, premedical, and predentistry. Before deciding on their major they work together, but even after a major has been declared they may continue to do so in some learning experiences. The point was made that such multidisciplinary teaching might be more successful if it begins at the preprofessional level.

The matrix model appears to have an inherent problem. Limiting the department chairman's role to career development tasks, clinical facilities development, and psychiatric residency training makes the chairmanship a less desirable post and thus more difficult to fill. Who will want the job when it becomes primarily administrative, assigning individuals to multidisciplinary teams where the teaching takes place, and persuading people to carry out organizational tasks? Such a chairman might be much less of a role model and more of a bureaucrat in this new system.

Finally, the point was made that in those schools where integrated or committee teaching has been tried, it provided the distinct advantage of not freezing the curriculum into a series of lectures and presentations on topics which are presented year after year. In spite of the burden on the faculty to attend organizational meetings, interdisciplinary teaching does provide constant evaluation, student input, and ease in changing courses in order to integrate findings from student and faculty evaluations.

The pros and cons of a separate behavioral sciences department were debated next. Resnik said that grouping the behavioral sciences together will prevent some of the identity problems of the nonphysician functioning in a medical school. As a department, behavioral scientists can have more influence on the curriculum as well as providing a common ground from which to operate. In a medical school, where they can easily be second-class citizens, to make them members of clinical departments may ensure that they have such status. A counter-point was made that since there are a variety of means for delivering educational objectives to students, medical schools may be organized in many different ways. Combining basic scientists with clinicians may, in fact, provide greater variability in medical schools than separate departments can; the problem may be that the non-M.D. teachers are concerned about their sense of identity and *want* to get together. So a behavioral science department might increase the possibility of providing better research in the delivery of health care, but not necessarily better learning experiences for students. Departments of behavioral science may be appropriate for some medical schools but not all, the reasons being totally unrelated to educational objectives for students.

Some schools that have tried the experiment of a separate department of behavioral sciences have had unhappy experiences. Often the basic scientists in such a department see themselves as predominantly research personnel rather than as clinical or educational people and are hesitant to contribute instruction. Also, this experiment leads to the false idea that the whole broad area of behavioral sciences, whether biological or psychosocial, can be incorporated under one department. The members of the various disciplines that deal with behavior are very different and do not get along as well together as one might hope. The separate department of behavioral sciences also creates some recruiting problems for the department of psychiatry since some psychiatrists are behavioral scientists as well as clinicians and teachers. A behavioral sciences department also tends to have a lower status in the eyes of students than departments in the "hard" basic sciences, such as physiology, microbiology, and biochemistry. In those schools where clinical departments are very strong, a weak behavioral science department may not do as well as a division of behavioral sciences under the umbrella of one or more clinical departments such as psychiatry or community medicine.

One unhappy experience occurred at the University of Oregon medical school, the first to have a separate department of medical psychology. The department was established more than ten years earlier on a tentative basis, to be reviewed after five years. At the end of that time it was decided the experiment was not successful, but the department was so entrenched that no change was possible. The difficulties are that the course program remains rather stereotyped and similar to a college major in psychology. More and more students have had courses in psychology and other behavioral sciences in college and consider the medical school courses redundant.

The participants seemed to feel that few separate departments of behavioral science have thus far been successful in terms of appeal to students, strong contributions to teaching, and ability to collaborate with psychiatry. On the other hand, some schools have had satisfactory or successful experiences with divisions of behavioral sciences within the department of psychiatry or with behavioral scientists in several departments of the medical school.

However, a minority opinion remained that the instructional objectives for medical students that relate to behavioral science can best be described and achieved by behavioral scientists and that their strongest base is to have their own department. This opinion was accompanied by the view that a behavioral science department failure, several of which had been described, really represented a failure of leadership on the part of the Dean who selected the chairman of the department of behavioral sciences.

A strong point was made that this discussion was not unlike that at meetings of professors of psychiatry for the past ten to fifteen years. But there are now many experiments going on with the numerous variables and issues that have been discussed over the years. For the first time several different models are being attempted for interdisciplinary teaching and matrix management and for the various ways of teaching behavioral science. It would be valuable to gather data from all the experiments over the next five to ten years and to see where they will be at the end of such a period. How will these medical schools evaluate their experiences in relation to what they are now doing and the fond hopes they express for the model they are attempting to implement?

Part Two

Residency Training
Programs

⋙⋙⋙⋙⋙⋙⋙⋙⋙⋙⋙⋙⋘⋘⋘⋘⋘⋘⋘⋘⋘⋘⋘⋘

Psychiatric residency training has generally followed the model of other postgraduate medical specialty training. The student has been rotated through a number of different clinical services. These vary with the nature of the institution sponsoring the training and often reflect service needs when that institution is a state hospital, a veterans' hospital, or a specialized university hospital. The student attends a few didactic conferences to gain a theoretical background, but the individual supervision approach is the foundation for clinical instruction. The student will be influenced by the orientation of his teacher.

Changes in the practice of psychiatry suggest corresponding changes in psychiatric training. The psychiatrist who used to be hospital-based or office-based is now likely to work with a mental health team, often in a community mental health center. These alterations necessitate reformulation of objectives in the education of the psychiatrist, of the type of setting in which he is trained, as well as the specific educational techniques and the clinical experiences necessary for training which will be relevant to his future practice and which will permit continued development in his professional life. Dr. Stubblefield organizes his own formulations from a background of years of experience as a psychiatry department chairman (Southwestern Medical School at Dallas) and as a leader in many organizations concerned with psychiatric education (such as the American Board of Psychiatry and Neurology); he is presently with the Western Interstate Commission on Higher Education. Dr. Shervington brings the experience of being chief of the Psychiatry Training Branch of the National Institute of Mental Health (NIMH).

3

Goals and Issues in Psychiatric Residency Training

ROBERT L. STUBBLEFIELD

*A*merican psychiatric education and training have been influenced by state hospitals, Veterans Administration hospitals, some of the leading private psychiatric hospitals, psychiatric services in general hospitals, university hospitals, neuropsychiatric institutes and, more recently, the community mental health centers. The quality of leadership has varied considerably, yet the general trend has been and is toward full-time academic and research-oriented leaders and away from program directors who engage exclusively in clinical practice.

Current planning suggests that general education is being influenced by a systems analysis approach, which permits one to assess a program in the areas of goals and objectives, planning and management of operational activities, and evaluation of outputs. In setting goals for a residency program in a medical school, many variables require consideration. Most will reflect the special interests and theoretical orientation of the psychiatry department in that medical school. Some departments are more interested in biological (bio-chemical) aspects of normal and disordered behavior; others pay special attention to the psychological forces influencing individual behavior (with a psychoanalytic or learning-theory orientation). A third group of programs focuses on psychosocial psychiatry and attends to interactional events rather than intrapsychic explanations. Many programs are eclectic and represent some combination of the other three.

Special qualities of the training program will be influenced by other factors. The age of the medical school will surely be one factor, because an established school with fixed traditions and lim-ited by older buildings will be different from the new school which has no traditions. The overall educational objectives of the medical school faculty, dean, and board of regents will also affect the psychi-atry program. Student competence varies among institutions. The clinical program carried on in a public charity hospital will be different from that in a private, nonprofit university hospital, a veterans' hospital, or a community mental health center. The avail-ability of research and teaching space and the adequacy of the bud-get are additional influences.

Using a program planning approach, one begins to tie insti-tutional goals into specific defined objectives for training a psychi-atrist. Two sets of factors then must be considered. First, personnel, space, and budget must be allocated properly and additional re-sources acquired if necessary to implement the objectives. Second, the expected results of a program must be estimated. If one hopes to graduate residents who will be teachers and research specialists, resources have to be carefully manipulated from the time residents are selected to the training process itself; a goal of producing eclectic clinicians requires teachers with certain beliefs and behavior.

Traditionally, the typical residency program divides into three activities: clinical care of patients; open, unscheduled time; and teaching conferences, rounds, seminars, and two to three hours of supervision per week. The clinical sequence has usually begun with inpatients, and the resident then moves to general hospital experiences, to outpatients and child psychiatry; much of the third year is quasi-independent work with less supervision and more responsibility for the resident to function as a consultant in mental health. This tradition now seems shattered, so that it is difficult to generalize about a typical program. Multiple clinical assignments, elective tracks, community assignments, and other new features have reshaped almost all programs. The greatest difficulty for the teacher is trying to predict the career choice of a resident. Many avenues are open, and the choice is often influenced by marriage, parenthood, personal therapy or analysis, special ego satisfactions in certain learning experiences, and the almost universal obligation for military service.

Finally, program directors and their faculties encounter problems in evaluating program effectiveness. Comparison with other residency programs is difficult. Results of the board examinations give some clues, but the data are often not available; the nature of the postresidency experience may shape or distort the residents' competence and skill considerably. For example, a busy private psychotherapeutic practice to pay off debts may destroy previously established study habits. A dispensary military assignment may alienate the young psychiatrist with research potential.

Variations in the type of residency program are influenced by a number of controversial issues in American psychiatry. The most striking, most debated, and least understood issue is the abolishment of the internship requirement. As I view the matter, this action was and is an attempt to face reality. The national effort to produce more physicians in a shorter time is evidenced in the acceptance of advanced students with two or three years of premedical work rather than four and in the federal capitation payments, which influence medical schools to graduate the student in three years rather than four.

Another problematic issue is the location of training. Some argue in favor of limited, concentrated efforts in a single hospital or service while others rotate residents through what seems to be an excessive number of casual service-oriented experiences. An additional area of controversy concerns the relationship between the theoretical orientation of the supervisor and the actual service responsibilities of the student. If his teacher is only interested in long-term individual psychotherapy and the student carries a large, crisis-oriented service responsibility, the conflict will cause difficulty. In such a situation the resident sees his training as irrelevant to the private psychotherapeutic practice he may wish to enter. The availability of related medical disciplines is a powerful argument for limiting residency training to medical school settings. However, this availability is often a paper promise, and in reality residents may not be encouraged to attend medical rounds or to keep abreast of modern developments in scientific medicine. Interaction between psychiatry and other medical specialties for learning purposes may occur more effectively in an affiliated program than in the caste system of a medical school.

I predict that future graduates will have to be trained in one of the twenty specialties or complete a military (or civilian) two-year assignment which will be supervised. I further predict that all physicians will have to be reexamined or certified for attendance in continuing education courses in order to maintain their right to practice medicine. Thus, the primary problem for the psychiatric training program director is to design a program that provides for the often-neglected component, namely, learning by identification over a significant period of time. I am optimistic that the present generation of students, who are healthier, better educated, less gullible than some previous generations, are capable of performing well in such a program.

There is great effort to maximize child psychiatric learning experiences in the general psychiatry residency. While I think it is constructive to teach about normal growth and development, to study families, and to study child psychopathology, I am skeptical about the goal of having every psychiatrist skilled in treating children. In a curious way, the community mental health movement has produced some practitioners who think that a few hours of therapy are enough for any crisis involving children. Others assume that anyone can play and talk with a child and that this interaction constitutes effective child therapy. My experience as a program director of treatment services for children does not bear these simplistic assumptions.

Interdisciplinary training is the great goal and dream of some of the NIMH staff. Not only should students of several disciplines be trained together, but they add that the training must be carried on by teachers from several disciplines. There is some unreality in this approach, perhaps even an unsubtle invasion of academic freedom. Most training directors want to build the self-awareness, self-esteem, and the individual diagnostic and treatment skills of the resident. The training director wants to help the young resident establish his professional identity and feeling of competence. Learning to work with interdisciplinary teams and to be taught by teachers of various disciplines can occur concurrently but should not be the dominant, overriding theme in the training program.

Psychoanalytic training remains the subject of a major controversy in American psychiatry. Although this training is not a fad, medical colleagues often view it in this manner. More and more departments evidence a hostile or indifferent attitude toward psychoanalysis, its values, and its contributions. Integration of psychoanalytic psychology into a residency program seems to depend, unfortunately, on personality factors in the academic community (the department and the psychoanalytic institute) and not enough on defined and discussed issues.

Neurology is another touchy subject. I think it is absurd for psychiatrists who deal with brain-mind-behavior issues to be indifferent to continued learning about the neurosciences. I deplore the attitude of a psychiatric resident who objects to a neurology learning experience and yet blithely dispenses psychotropic drugs as if he were a competent neurophysiologist. By the same token, some neurologists refuse to teach psychiatrists and retreat into departments of medicine (where there is money, power, and patients who are covered by third-party payments).

I subscribe to the efforts to have psychiatric residents learn a great deal about minorities and their problems, although I do not believe psychiatrists have many answers to the racism issue. I argue for concentration on an area that is accessible, with teachers who are knowledgeable, rather than multiple, rapid rotations through many services and locations in the community for the sake of exposure to a variety of ethnic subcultures.

A final issue is examinations. In order for medical schools to be leaders in training psychiatrists they should be involved in regular assessment of residents' performances and skills. The medical school must be active in sharing observations about gaps and deficiencies in a resident's performance and should not be content with simply recording levels of competence for future letters of reference.

Training for
Community Service

WALTER W. SHERVINGTON

अ अ अ अ अ अ अ अ अ अ अ अ अ अ ᒃ ᒃ ᒃ ᒃ ᒃ ᒃ ᒃ ᒃ ᒃ ᒃ ᒃ

Since the beginning of the NIMH after World War II, psychiatry has moved steadily, although slowly, in the direction of attempting to serve communities. The first communities served were the private-practice community and the university, since previously there had been insufficient manpower in the mental health professions. Now we face the task of serving large and complex communities, which is by no means an easy chore and involves more than providing direct services such as psychotherapy, behavior therapy, drug therapy, and somatic therapies. If psychiatry is ultimately to make these therapies available to all people in need, if we are going to approach alcoholism, drug addiction, psychoses, neuroses, racism, senility, and organic illnesses as they affect people in communities, then training a psychiatrist exclusively in individual psychotherapy will poorly equip him to face the task ahead. This model of individual interaction between psychiatrist and patient or psychiatrist and group must change. Some of us fear a loss of income and status from such a change, yet psychiatrists in community work continue to earn reasonable salaries plus fringe benefits and may still have some private practice income. Psychiatrists who are good in community work continue to have elevated status, though not necessarily within the training institutions. I am not denigrating psychotherapeutic work with patients but raising a question about its position in our training. The training of a psychiatrist is too broad, or at least it should be, and much too costly to have him serve so few. The problems that we face from the standpoint of health and social illness are much too great not to have maximum psychiatric input and participation in their resolution.

We must recognize that the role of the physician, the practice of medicine, the cost of medical care, and who gets that care are presently under scrutiny. Psychiatry is no exception. Some colleagues have already spoken of difficulties in maintaining an individual psychotherapy practice. They do not feel this phenomenon is related purely and simply to the overabundance of psychiatrists in some urban areas, but perhaps is a result of an increasingly sophisticated public in those areas. This public perhaps no longer believes it must pay top dollar for psychiatric care, clearly feeling that it can obtain psychotherapy from other mental health professionals or that group therapy will work as well as individual treatment. In brief, the public is questioning the validity of the old model. The more we reject leadership in the broad field of mental health, the greater is the basis for that view.

How should we train people to work within communities? The best place to do that training is within the community. But I do not mean simply placing a resident in the community. Young psychiatrists should be in an environment that maximizes the delivery of public service to those in need more than one which emphasizes individual enterprise. We cannot train a man to be an individual entrepreneur, encourage him to work within a system where he is to be top dog, not working in concert with others, and then expect him to leave that training program and adequately serve a community. If a psychiatric resident begins his training with a broad approach, learning that he must understand individuals and the community in order to deliver service, he will have a different level of consciousness from that of the trainee in most programs today. All residents in the country do not have to be trained in precisely the same way. Diversity of curriculum because of the enrichment it affords must remain. And not every psychiatrist ought to be a generalist; but, whatever his specialty in psychiatry, he should have the skills developed by this broad approach.

How can such a training experience be implemented, while at the same time enabling the trainee to develop an identity as a psychiatrist? One suggestion is that the first year, instead of being spent on the traditional inpatient service, be spent at a community mental health center (or a community service if a center is not available) where the resident is a member of a team responsible for a catchment area. He should be encouraged to see patients in their immediate communities, with families, friends, or in community agencies. He can learn about and develop an understanding of individual dynamics, group dynamics, and family dynamics within this framework. In fact he can better understand individual dynamics if he is forced to look beyond the individual patient to the family and the influences of the various forces within a community. Clearly, the needs of training take precedence over the needs of service because of the new demands on the psychiatrist to broaden his expertise and functioning. Residents should deliver service only to the extent that they thereby develop an understanding of their responsibility to give service.

For the resident to have the intensive and broad experiences outlined, the director of residency training must indeed earn his money. In the past the director had to be concerned that his residents had sufficient numbers of long-term individual psychotherapy cases with psychoneurotic, somatic, and psychotic illnesses, along with a certain amount of group therapy experience. Now he has a few additional learning situations to provide, but the task is not impossible. He should be sure they see both male and female training models from a variety of ethnic backgrounds; they should be able to interview, diagnose, and evaluate children and adults; they should be able to work psychotherapeutically in groups and with families; they should be able to work with people from other disciplines; and they should be able to consult with agencies and use agencies in the treatment of patients. Didactic instruction in psychotherapy, behavioral approaches, human development, community approaches, and community consultation must also be a part of such a training program. Since in the United States racial and ethnic struggles are so much a part of the daily lives of all of us, the trainee should gain insight into these struggles through courses taught by competent persons.

Training in the skills of psychotherapy for both adults and children can take place simultaneously. Residents can carry cases in long-term psychotherapy, short-term psychotherapy, brief psychotherapy, crisis intervention, family and group psychotherapy throughout their training. Such experiences do not all have to happen at once, yet they do not either have to be divided into a block system, which is unnatural to the occurrence of illness within the community. Training by a block system is destined to create a psychiatrist who is never able to get the total picture and must, as a result, resort to treating in a very piecemeal fashion, always on his own terms, and more often than not in the isolation of his office. Care must be taken in developing training programs not only to encourage the resident to be a social activist but also to ensure that social action becomes a part of his therapeutic armamentarium.

Let us turn now to some of the specific issues facing residency training. To begin, imagine what might be the case if the funding pattern changes and the psychiatric residency training support comes through the Health Maintenance Organization (HMO) and third-party payment systems. If at the same time funding for the outreach and consultative activities of community mental health centers is phased out, the psychiatrist will be forced to limit his activities to those that fall within the confines of the medical model—that is, activities related to the diagnosis, evaluation, and treatment of functional or organic psychiatric illnesses or both. Our consultation with other medical specialties will continue, and perhaps our understanding of cultural, ethnic, and racial struggles will continue to be important, especially as they relate to the resolution of psychiatric illness. However, the consultative activities, the outreach activities, those activities which attempt to approach mental illness at its root and to develop sophisticated primary preventative methods, will have to be abandoned because of insufficient funding resources. The most distinct dangers of the HMO legislation as presently proposed are that it will put the focus back on inpatient beds and leave no support for preventive measures. However, it is early in the legislative process and change is still possible. Psychiatry must point out the need for support of indirect services. Also competition between HMOs might create the necessity to develop indirect services in order to increase the profit margin of any one HMO. I am not convinced, however, that the latter would be allowed to happen.

Consider next how the loss of the internship for psychiatrists might affect them in practice. Many fear that the sense of responsibility that is and should be supreme in medical practice will be lessened. They feel that participating in the birth and death experiences is very significant to the character of the physician. If this view is correct, and most likely it is, perhaps such responsibility can be preserved by building into the first year a very rigorous experience that gives the young psychiatrist responsibility for the quality of life of his patients and community and that provides work with the dying patient.

Consider still a different question: the integration of psychoanalytic training into basic residency training. Psychodynamics remain essential to the core curriculum in the psychotherapy segment of psychiatric training. Intensive understanding of the psychoanalytic approach clearly can do nothing but enhance greatly the understanding of individual psychodynamics and broaden the availability of the psychiatric trainee. And if the trainee enters a personal analysis, he may be freed from those individual conflicts which might interfere with the breadth of his training.

However, psychoanalysis continues to be a form of treatment for the wealthy few because of the amount of time, energy, and money that must go into it. There is also some question as to whether psychoanalysis can serve the needs of other than the well-to-do intellectual, not because of the nature of the problems experienced by those others but because of the problems inherent in psychoanalytic training and practice: the seeming unwillingness of most practitioners to adequately take account of racial, cultural, and ethnic data; the severe hierarchy that has always existed in psychoanalytic circles and which creates an atmosphere antithetical to well-grounded training in a community setting; and the continuing and ever-present secrecy that seems to accompany psychoanalytic deliberations and psychoanalysts, be that truly the case or not. The continuing elevated status of the private practicing psychoanalyst and his influence in psychoanalytic institutes would clearly mitigate against the development of the consciousness of public service desired in the trainee in a community center.

Psychoanalysis and psychoanalytic education must continue to flourish, as they are still important contributors to a theoretical understanding of individual psychology. But there is ample room for improvement. (As Robert Cohen so frequently says, "Psychoanalytic theory is not a very good theory, but it is probably the best theory of individual psychology that we have.") As much as many progressive psychoanalysts would like to make psychoanalytic training available earlier and would like to graduate younger psychoanalysts, with the recognition of the use of psychoanalytic understanding in a context other than the private practice/private office model, the hazards of such early training still appear much greater than the possible assets. Those who are going to use their psychoanalytic training in its broadest context, in the service of the community as well as in the service of the individual, will most likely do so even if such training is acquired as part of late residency or postresidency education.

Another issue concerns the electives and multifaceted approaches in our residency programs. These are increasing in number. Theoretically, because of increasing elective schedules, a resident might pass through the program without ever learning the techniques of psychotherapy and perhaps even the techniques of diagnosis and evaluation. But some programs are so closed that the newer and "more radical" approaches to patient care or to communities are never experienced or investigated. One appears to be too loose and one too rigid. We need to decide on a core curriculum which will be broader than the previous one (which was based primarily on psychodynamic understanding). Then we should allow maximal opportunity to complete the core curriculum within the first two years. The third year can be elective or track. With the many subspecialties now developing in psychiatry, there is clearly a need for specialization, which can be attained through the third-year elective and track system (adding a fourth year) without sacrificing the basic and core knowledge. Such a program is particularly possible since many students will come to the psychiatric residency with increased psychiatric sophistication as a result of their electives in the fourth year of medical school. However, let us not be obsessed with the idea that the core curriculum must precede electives. Elective time may come at the beginning. Perhaps most important is to decide on a core curriculum and leave the time for its absorption to the trainee.

Multiple tracks must be encouraged in order to ensure sufficient training of some students in specific or subspecialty areas. However, multiple tracks should not be encouraged simply to bring new monies into training programs. Courses which should be included in basic training or in basic components of subspecialty training should not be deferred in order to keep them in a special training program.

There has been considerable discussion about the benefits of interdisciplinary training. Such training would make the psychiatrist a better psychiatrist, the psychologist a better psychologist, the nurse a better nurse, and the social worker a better social worker. Many of us who were trained several years ago are increasingly aware of our wishes for increased knowledge of and experience in the other disciplines. Two advantages, among others, of interdisciplinary training immediately appear attractive. One is enhancement of the individual's understanding by broadening his training, and the other the possibility that interdisciplinary collaboration can increase appreciation for other disciplines. I hope some of both will be accomplished when training truly takes place in the community setting, with people of several disciplines being taught by an interdisciplinary faculty those aspects of the curriculum that are common to all. Interdisciplinary training of mental health specialists who plan administrative, public health, or academic careers could now be a subspecialty elective or track for the psychiatrist. In the future, perhaps most psychiatric training will be interdisciplinary.

Research training of psychiatrists must also be encouraged, perhaps in the first two years with small projects that would not demand so much attention as to take away from the core curriculum. Intensive training could begin in the third year as a research track.

Much that I have discussed could progress with continued support at the present level and higher, along with responsible administration at NIMH, which I am hopeful the Psychiatry Training Branch will be able to deliver. The narrow approach to training and limiting the activities of the psychiatrist would be, in my view, most unfortunate at this time. Alexander H. Leighton (1971), head of the Department of Behavioral Sciences, Harvard School of Public Health, discussing the high "symptoms of psychiatric disorders" and their impact on societal structures, states, "The resultant pathology can take many shapes and spread far much like a contagious disease." Leighton concludes that if we are to avoid "prejudice, environmental destruction, overpopulation, and nuclear war, then the psychiatrist will have to join with other disciplines to bring experience and knowledge to bear on the crucial issues of our times."

Discussion

The flow of the discussion related to the position papers by Stubblefield and Shervington highlighted several key issues, particularly the problem of redefinition of core curriculum and core experience in psychiatric residency training. This task is made more difficult because we appear to be at a crossroads: in one direction a traditional medical orientation to psychiatric training, in the other a preventive-social-community orientation. There is clearly more than one kind of psychiatrist being trained today, and the possibility of multitrack approaches was considered—that is, what kinds of elective specialized experiences should be offered during residency training? Finally, the community mental health orientation of the newer departments of psychiatry relates to the issues of interdisciplinary training for mental health professionals and requires discussion of the settings and service models within which the training occurs. The "politics" involved in service and training combinations will be a main topic of subsequent chapters. This section presents major subtopics and the principal alternative points of view surrounding them, as they were discussed by the participants.

Psychodynamic Psychotherapy

While exposure to psychotherapy may continue to be important for all trainees, it is unrealistic today to think residents in a three-year period can become expert in this form of psychotherapy. Perhaps one of four trainees will end up as psychotherapists, and the development of their definitive skills in psychotherapy continues in the next several years beyond their three-year training period. The intensive psychoanalytic model seems to have given way to the broader community model as the magnetic force in residency training. Psychoanalytic treatment remains the treatment for the very few and therefore a psychoanalytic institute within a department of psychiatry may be antithetical to a community-oriented training program.

New Components of Core Experience

Child psychiatry must be further integrated as part of general psychiatry training. Most psychiatrists are dealing with children and adolescents through consultation work or direct therapy, short- or long-term. However, it is questionable whether all general psychiatrists can become as competent diagnostic and treatment experts with children as with adults, since there are some who just cannot interact as effectively with children.

Neurosciences are increasingly crucial. Even if neurology and psychiatry should split into separate "boards," the psychiatrist-to-be must know about brain behavior as well as the community. Other important categories are alcoholism and drug abuse. Competence in these areas also involves the psychiatrist in the community and require the ability to work with teams of other professionals, paraprofessionals, and community representatives. And experience with the problems of different ethnic and minority groups is also becoming essential. Trainees can probably learn about the necessity for understanding the various groups by working in one such supervised experience.

Traditionally, psychiatrists have been taught that they were "finished" in three years—that the core was enough in itself to complete a psychiatrist. With the present half-life of medical knowledge so short, we now realize that one must be trained to continue studying indefinitely. The danger in defining core is structuring it as final rather than as a continuing process. Relicensing and recertification will undoubtedly be incorporated into medicine, and psychiatrists will either be reexamined or show other evidence of being up to date in the field.

Because of the "crossroads" phenomenon and the difficulty of defining psychiatry core functions in the future, it is possible to look at psychiatry as a multitrack specialty. There is no longer a single kind of psychiatrist. Enelow's group has identified the following kinds: (1) general clinical psychiatrist; (2) child psychiatrist; (3) psychotherapist-psychoanalyst; (4) group or family psychotherapist; (5) consultation or liaison psychiatrist; (6) academic psychiatrist; (7) academic-research psychiatrist; (8) administrative-managerial psychiatrist; (9) politician. Perhaps programs should choose several of these models which they might be able to reasonably accomplish successfully. Those that produce hard-core, one-to-one therapists and nothing else should be known for excellence in that field, whereas those who produce social change experts should be known as well for their characteristics.

Sequences of Clinical Experience

Drug addiction, alcoholism and children's problems are examples of important new experiences. The question is when to start them and for how long in the newer rotations. Some find that if you do not start them early as part of a comprehensive mental health training experience the resident has difficulty becoming involved later. On the other hand, many feel that development of basic diagnostic and treatment skills must occur in a closely supervised situation to provide the basic identity for a psychiatrist, that is, the traditional sequence of resident experience—the hospital inpatient service and outpatient clinic in the first year or two of training. The community outreach experience is then added later.

Some programs are finding that immersion in a community outreach program is the best way to start residency training. The model most frequently used is that of the interdisciplinary team which has responsibility for delivering care to a certain defined population with the hope that most of the mental health issues in the community will come to that team. Thus a resident, while working with the team, will have an opportunity to begin working with a family and evaluating a child in that family. He would also be able to pick up cases from that community to begin the process of long-term intensive psychotherapy. It requires a good deal of planning and work by the program director to make sure a resident has a variety of experiences and can integrate them to help him evolve his skills as a psychiatrist.

Psychiatry is now more than simply the treatment of mental illness but also a tool for social change: the community model has been added to the medical model. Programming for our nation covers more than what is in the diagnostic manual, with a broader mission than the treating of psychopathological conditions; thus, the mental health concept is replacing the mental illness concept. The newer models of training experience point up the commonalities which are not unique to psychiatry. Should we design a system to include all mental health disciplines, professions, and subprofessions that are going to be involved? If they are going to work together we should think of training them in the same classroom and clinical setting and perhaps even giving them the same supervisory experience.

Community-Oriented Interdisciplinary Training

Identity diffusion is a problem in the developing psychiatrist. At some time the resident needs to interact with the supervisor without a cluster of people around him. Just as the man who operates and finds an inoperable tumor cannot discuss in the presence of thirty to fifty technical people the dilemmas which lead him to his decision to close the patient, so the psychiatrist needs to have some intimate one-to-one learning experiences as a physician-to-be. Training which is completely interdisciplinary from beginning to end in which one never gets an opportunity to meet one's role model would not produce a psychiatrist as we presently know him.

The critical mass problem is another issue. Can you train a psychiatrist for his entire three years in a community mental health center if that program does not supply the values involved in research and high-quality education and if nobody is specifically assigned to do at least half-time teaching? You can use the delivery-of-service model for education if you have the critical mass of manpower and if you have enough control of the center to combine and blend the service and educational functions. Residents should not be placed in centers with no one there to supervise them and to help with the struggles they will face. If there is a teacher who is either a liaison from the faculty or a part-center and part-faculty person, this model is more likely to succeed.

Most agree that there is no incompatibility between developing basic clinical competence and ability to work in a community mental health center. Students can be placed on a team that serves a catchment area and protected from too many demands by having a large enough faculty who are good role models and who are involved in the delivery of services. One may also have to help the resident with his own anxiety of not knowing who he is by taking him out of the interdisciplinary group at times as he cements his identity, but he must have the capacity to approach a clinical problem in the context of the multiplicity of factors and agencies involved in the community. The mixing and blending of the faculty of an academic department in a community mental health center allows for the running of a comprehensive clinical service in addition to teaching and training. Identification is a very basic part of learning.

Funding

Historically, NIMH has always funded "communities" in one way or another. First were the academic and private practice communities, quite necessary to bulid to have a critical mass before a mental health impact could be made on the medical society. Now the community being supported is the "general" community, and mental health professionals are trained for a broad context. As a result, funds seem to be shifting to support training staff for community mental health centers and to service certain critical problem categories, such as alcohol and drug abuse.

National health insurance appears more and more likely, and the funding of psychiatric services is a minor part of it. At the same time community mental health center funding is being threatened.

We may find ourselves training psychiatrists principally for providing care with an HMO. The psychiatrist would be trained to do direct diagnosis and treatment almost exclusively for this system, a rather limited role compared to that available in the present community mental health development.

Thus it is difficult to design a core curriculum because we cannot be sure at this point whether the psychiatrist of the seventies is going to be identified more with the medical HMO model or with the social community model. The HMO model would cut back on community outreach orientation, consultation and prevention, basically training psychiatrists to work in medical settings. On the other hand, if community mental health funding continues to grow, we will probably move further toward "mental health specialists," among whom psychiatrists will be one group. The disciplines—psychiatry, social work, psychology, nursing, and so on—will come to an interdisciplinary focus with a certain kind of background attitude that remains important for all of them.

Part Three

New Settings

≋≋≋≋≋≋≋≋≋≋≋≋≋≋≋≋≋≋≋≋≋≋≋≋≋≋≋≋

Some readers will wince at the topic of new settings, expecting a catalog-like idealized description of physical facilities. Instead, our intent is to focus on the hard realities which relate the clinical setting to the educational program; for to a greater degree than most dare admit the setting determines the design and the effectiveness of the educational program.

We appear to be at a critical point in the shift from small inpatient hospital settings, which focus on quality control and teaching but occupy a too-large slice of the resident's time, to the catchment-area concept that emphasizes ambulatory care and a natural occurrence of various human problems but can be so overwhelmed by enormous service demands that quality care is jeopardized. Some of the most traditional schools have already been left behind, frozen into old models, while some of the newer schools are already involved with new experiments whose problems they did not anticipate. However, most new schools have their options open and are struggling with how to balance interlocking educational and service issues and their role in the delivery of both. Dr. Romano, long recognized as one of the foremost psychiatric medical educators in the country, distills the best of the traditional point of view and urges us to preserve the hospital as a modern version of the complete educational setting. Dr. Webster, as director of the Continuing

Education Branch of the National Institute of Mental Health, has, over the past few years, ranged across the nation visiting a wide variety of programs and has noted the congruities and incongruities between the dual functions of education and service.

5

Clinical Settings for
Educational Programs

JOHN ROMANO

*W*hat does *clinical setting* mean?
Is it restricted to the description and dimensions of physical space,
of basic architectural design, or does it refer to the general intellectual and political ambience of the university, the medical school,
or the hospital in which the space may be sought? Does it refer to
the general availability of professional and paraprofessional personnel? Should it include some relation to the community in which the
educational program is conducted? Obviously, the clinical setting
must be a place where the essential trinity of the patient, the student,
and the teacher can meet and become engaged in a common venture.

Criteria for the optimal setting will depend on who is to be
taught (whether he be medical student, nursing student, psychology
and social work student, psychiatric resident, social science student,
paraprofessional). Furthermore, the criteria will be affected not
only by those to be taught but by what they are to be taught, and

for what purpose. What are the objectives of the several educational programs?

I have taken the liberty of posting these caveats as I firmly believe that the clinical setting, in its broadest connotative sense, derives from a host of other factors, the essence of which includes the amount of information and technology available, the transmissibility of the available information and technology, and the value that society places on the available information and technology, which in turn is based on the social and economic structure of that society. In what follows, I pay particular attention to the medical student, although much applies equally to the education of the psychiatric resident.

The current trend in medical education, if it continues, may significantly affect the clinical setting of the several educational programs. If the professional educational period of the medical student is reduced from four to three years, and the free-standing internship eliminated or woven into a truncated graduate resident period, there will be a loss of two years, occurring at a most strategic moment in the maturation of the clinician. These are the two years usually considered to be phase-specific for learning the physician's role. On other occasions and in earlier papers I have discussed these matters in detail (Romano, 1963, 1964, 1968, 1970a, 1970b).

Wherever the trends may take us and our students, will tomorrow's students enjoy the opportunities that today's students have to learn about mental illness? In a recent paper (Romano, 1972), I said that today's student studies and cares for the mentally sick patient in the same hospital setting in which he studies and cares for other patients. The establishment of psychiatric services in general teaching hospitals, together with the development of full- and part-time clinical faculties, have made this possible. The student becomes aware of the perplexity, despair, confusion, anxiety, shame, and guilt of the mentally ill patient and learns of the impact of the illness on members of the patient's family. He learns why much of mental illness has been taught to be due to magic and sorcery and to supernatural factors and how recent are the attempts to understand human behavior in naturalistic terms. As he grows in his new role of clinician, he learns of the effectiveness as well as the limitations of emergency, short-term, and long-term hospital care;

of psychotherapeutic attitudes as exhibited by himself and by others in the care of the patient; of the use of psychotropic drugs; and of the dramatic success of ECT with depressed patients. He learns of the multiple set, that there are many who share with him the study and care of the sick, and that he must identify and differentiate his role from those of his associates. He learns, too, that the patient is also a member of a group, of a family, and of other groups, and that the patient's behavior cannot be understood clearly if dealt with in isolation.

Throughout the teaching hospital, in its several clinical divisions and in his various assignments—inpatient, outpatient, emergency—and more recently in extramural neighborhood health centers the student learns of the psychology and sociology of the patient. He learns about them as the patient experiences acute or chronic illness, and he will also learn of the special psychosocial problems of the handicapped, the chronic psychotic, the deformed, the retarded, the epileptic, the blind, and the deaf. The general hospital settings also provides opportunity for studying patients with intractable pain, in which evidence of structural impairment is minimal; patients with disparate convalescent patterns in which recovery from injury, illness, and surgical intervention has been surprisingly rapid or unduly delayed; patients with nonspecific symptoms of fatigue, restlessness, irritability, depression, insomnia, or bereavement.

A third opportunity lies in the concern with methods of observation. As David Shakow has told us, the student learns the distinctions between objective observation, participant observation, subjective observation, and self-observation. He learns that this differentiation is central to understanding the patient-physician relationship, in which the student's role depends on and emerges from his basic capacity for human intimacy.

The student learns of the general notion of personality and the basic principles which underly this understanding: genic and ontogenetic factors in growth, development, and decline; the recognition of unconscious and preconscious factors as determinants of behavior; the notion of drive-derivative behavior; the idea that the personality is integral and indivisible; the psychosocial principle which recognizes that man is a social animal and that the emerging stages of the life cycle must be understood in terms of the crucial coordination between the developing individual and his social environment. And this dual study of biology and personality has led to a clearer concept of health and disease and to the realization that psychopathology survives, and regretfully prospers, under many flags. The fallacy of the single cause is nowhere more obvious than in considerations of health and disease.

These, then, are several of the opportunities today's students have. I believe them to be substantial contributions to the education of the physician and that psychiatry has played a significant part in their achievement. Are tomorrow's students to have these opportunities? Most of the contributions have taken place in the territory of the psychiatric unit of the general hospital. For this reason, the medical student and the career psychiatric resident have had less experience with certain groups of patients, who, for several reasons, do not come to the general hospital or are discouraged or prohibited from coming. These include the chronic psychotic, except at points of crisis; the addict, including the alcoholic; the delinquent and criminal; the aged; and the psychotic and brain-damaged child. Many of these patients are seen in the emergency division, in outpatient visits, and in short-term inpatient stays, but few, for obvious reasons, can be studied or cared for for longer periods of time in the general hospital. In these matters we are no different from our medical and surgical colleagues, who must transfer chronically ill patients to other health services. Historically and traditionally the halls of academic medicine have never been associated with the care of chronic illness except for rare research ventures. The amount of useful, practical, and transmissible information and technology concerning much of chronic illness is limited. Chronic illness, more than acute illness, carries with it many issues of poverty, housing, unemployment—matters about which most physicians have acquired little information beyond that which they have learned as general citizens.

If medical education is to become seriously engaged in the study and care of certain groups of patients, currently seen in limited fashion, this involvement may lead to broader consortiums of health service facilities to which students will be assigned. May I add a word of caution. If the student is to be moved away from the central teaching hospital—to the chronic hospital, to the neighborhood health center, to the drug abuse first-aid center, to schools and courts—I believe it most important that he be assigned to and supervised by an experienced, informed, and committed senior professional person with whom the student may find it possible to identify. Incidentally, for those of you who believe, like Santayana, that those who forget the past may be condemned to repeat it, I draw your attention to the historical fact that our psychiatric colleagues and predecessors over many years have been concerned with the physical setting of teaching. In the broadest sense of teaching, as a professional group we have been publicly more concerned about our teaching habits than has any other professional group with which I have become acquainted. In 1912 the Association of American Medical Colleges conducted a survey of psychiatric teaching. There was another in 1914 by W. W. Graves, in 1933 by R. A. Noble, and in 1942 by Franklin Ebaugh and Charles Rymer. We are far more gregarious than de Tocqueville thought possible. The first conference on psychiatric education was in 1933, the second in 1934, the third in 1935, and the fourth in 1936. There was a wartime conference, supported by the Commonwealth Fund in 1945, and the famous Ithaca Conferences took place in 1951 and 1952. The World Health Organization of the United Nations conducted a world survey in 1962, and there was another American conference in Atlanta in 1967. Each meeting produced a sizable, and occasionally readable, report. (Ebaugh, 1942, 1944; Graves, 1914; Noble, 1933; American Psychiatric Association, 1969; World Health Organization, 1961). Perhaps we are more concerned with teaching or more anxious or less secure or more lonely than we were in the past. Whatever the reasons, we seem to need to meet with each other often. One can learn a great deal from the reports of the surveys and conferences. In reports almost forty years old one can find good accounts of some of the special problems of teaching in outpatient departments, state hospitals, state schools, and liaison teaching on medical, surgical, and pediatric floors of a general hospital. As is well known, the greatest degree of success in promoting teaching occurred after the two Ithaca Conferences (American Psychiatric Association, 1952, 1953). Whatever success followed these conferences depended in great part on what preceded them, but there was one difference that distinguished them from previous ventures. The Ithaca Conferences and the recommendations that ensued from them were generously nourished by federal funds, available for the development of both undergraduate and graduate teaching programs. So far as I know, this support had no precedent. Its success reinforces a point I made earlier: even when there is sufficient transmittable information and technology available, it is also necessary that society consider their transmission sufficiently valuable to support it.

From our experience and after a number of experiments with other systems, I remain convinced that the central, most important and useful assignment for the medical student in his first clinical year is to the inpatient psychiatric service in the general teaching hospital for a reasonable period of time, not less than six or more than eight weeks. Here the student has time to become involved with his patient and his patient's family. He can see at first hand and participate in the interdisciplinary work of patient care. There is continuity of observation, adequate supervision of his work, and provisions to lessen his initial anxiety in dealing with the mad. With this experience at hand, the student can acquire the emotional and intellectual confidence and competence to deal with anxious, upset, depressed, paranoid persons wherever he may meet them, in school, home, factory, outpatient department, on the medical floors of the hospital, in the neighborhood health center, or in his office, whether he be alone or with a group. I hope we can continue to provide our students with this experience, which makes possible the mastery of the phase-specific task of becoming a clinician—namely, the disciplining of his capacity for human intimacy.

In sum, my position is close to that of President Garfield when he said, "I am not willing that this discussion should close without mention of the value of a true teacher. Give me a log hut, with only a simple bench, Mark Hopkins on one end and I on the other, and you may have all the buildings, apparatus, and libraries without him."

Planning and Implementing
New Strategies

Thomas G. Webster

ƻƻƻƻƻƻƻƻƻƻƻƻƻƻƙƙƙƙƙƙƙƙƙƙƙƙƙƙ

New medical schools have great opportunity and freedom to consider thoughtfully their institutional goals and educational program objectives *and then* to tailor clinical settings which are most congruent with those goals and objectives. Classically, the nature of the training facilities has strongly determined the nature of the program, and this is inevitable to some degree. The influences of the setting are obvious in many respects; yet over time so much gets "built into the woodwork" that the influences on program may become quite subtle. In my observation the inhabitants of a given setting often have some culture-blindness about such effects. For example, when the facilities are heavily weighted by large inpatient units with a heavy case load, faculty members are apt to argue the merits and have an elaborate educational rationale for why inpatient work provides the best training. The same is true for those who occupy a given university hospital, child guidance clinic, or community mental health center.

Despite such adaptive but narrowing human tendencies,

much can be done to make clinical settings more relevant to program objectives. One might consider the education program first and then adapt the setting to the objectives. Examples of schools which established their program first are the Medical College of Ohio at Toledo, the East Virginia Medical School, and Pennsylvania State University at Hershey. Another alternative is to develop conceptual and functional freedom from the constraints and biases imposed by any given facilities. One means is to increase the faculty's awareness of the many ways the setting influences the program. Sometimes this awareness is enhanced by visiting other training centers; the contrasts help sharpen faculty perceptions.

Continuing commitment to the educational objectives and periodic review of the influences of the setting are important in any training setting. Observers from outside as well as inside the system can help provide a balanced perspective. One can invite visits by outside faculty, as well as arrange for visits to other schools by new department chairmen and key faculty members. NIMH review committees and staff are another resource to consult about establishing programs and settings. The fact that faculty members move from one school to another obviously makes available certain additional information to those planning new settings. And some schools have found faculty retreats to be valuable. A faculty away from the pressures of telephones and clinical responsibilities can plan more creatively. Other resources include conferences of psychiatric educators, such as the various professors' meetings.

Determining institutional or organizational goals and specifying educational program objectives are technical processes. Expert consultants can help facilitate planning. Representatives of key groups with a vested interest in the outcome should participate such as administrators, faculty, trainees, practitioners, employers of graduates, consumers of services). Information on existing manpower and patterns of practice can serve as a baseline for planning and as a basis for future evaluation.

The planning group must consider the institutional charter and mandate and must become familiar with the legal responsibilities originating therefrom. Informal determinants such as historical, economic, and political factors must also be considered. The group must ask: does the institutional purpose support a psychiatric education program and what are the realistic limitations and constraints?

The faculty must also consider whom the institution was created to serve. What population base or community are the trainees being prepared to serve? A department of psychiatry may define a particular population as the "laboratory setting" for training, research, and services. If the problems and principles of this training setting are learned well, graduates are better prepared to assess the uniqueness of any future setting in which they may work. Epidemiology, case registers, market research, consumer spokesmen, and other sources of information provide the basis for determining health service priorities and strategies. The university should utilize available data and become a contributor of future data, participating collaboratively in consortia of government and private agencies in the cyclical planning and evaluation process. Program objectives of the psychiatry department for the defined population can thus be determined with awareness of other resources and clinical settings which serve the same population. Examples of schools using this approach to planning include the University of Hawaii and the University of Rochester.

Manpower development and training program objectives can be determined in the context of the laboratory setting. Faculty and students should thus become aware of how physicians, psychiatrists, and the students themselves fit into the picture of human resources available to the defined population. All mental health training programs in the area should be considered in planning the specific objectives and role of the psychiatry training programs. This picture has a conceptual base that is gradually concretized in clinical settings and their interdisciplinary training functions. Two schools which have considered how their services fit into the overall picture of human resources available in their areas are the State University of New York at Stony Brook and the East Carolina University.

Concrete education program objectives are developed according to level of training, types of trainees, and circumstances of a given year. Interdisciplinary training, including paraprofessionals and new careerists, should be dovetailed with discipline-specific and level-specific training. Thoughtful attention should be given to teamwork functions and professional identity formation for all disciplines.

Building location, space relations, and architecture can facilitate or impede these learning and developmental process—more accurately, they help shape the products of the educational program. The faculty must ask whether the clinical setting is shaping trainees to fit the past, the present, or the future. Planning interdisciplinary training has occurred at the University of Missouri at Kansas City, the University of Texas at San Antonio, and the University of Southern California.

Epidemiologic and social science research should be developed in the "community" laboratory setting, which consists of specific populations. Contributions of other schools and departments of the university can be integrated most successfully when all are working in the same community laboratory. Economics, law, political science, child development, education, biological behavioral sciences, and clinical research can be most naturally related to health and psychiatric program objectives in such a setting. Examples here might include Michigan State University, the University of California at Davis, and Tufts University.

In order to implement a program, planners must consider at least four aspects of the clinical setting. First, the physical surroundings, including geographic features of the community and neighborhood, should be examined. The physical environment must obviously be appropriate for mental health programs as well as education. Transportation for clients must be considered. The design of any building would depend on advance study of traffic flow and of activity and work groupings. Planners should also determine whether all services can be centralized in a single unit or whether there should be outreach programs from some type of home base. The educational program will require technology and equipment of its own, including communication systems, study space for students, and laboratories.

A second aspect is the organizational structure. The organization may include a constellation of hospitals, clinics, community agencies, and schools as well as consortia of various training programs. Certainly funding patterns for construction and for the establishment of service and training must be considered. Professional societies and influential practitioners must also be involved in the educational program as advisors and teachers. The organization will also be concerned with legislation, advisory groups, and citizen participation.

The third consideration is how to design the setting for direct patient care. What must be delineated is the selection process for patients and accessibility for patients and other clients. Psychiatry and mental health programs must be related tangibly and physically to comprehensive health settings. There must also be collaboration among a variety of resource persons as part of the everyday work in the clinical setting. Alternatives must be provided for the patient and family within a context of continuity of care. A mental health program will be concerned with prevention as well as direct treatment activities. The treatment offered must include a range of appropriate types, including biological, psychological, and social approaches. Research activities must be relevant to biopsychosocial aspects of patient care.

Final consideration must be given to educational needs. Education in such a clinical program must be a daily way of life and there must be built-in and environmental stimuli for the learner. Precautions must be taken that the lessons learned are consistent with the intended instruction. Educational programs must provide access to faculty and to peer groups. Instructors and role models must be visibly engaged in work the trainees are expected to learn. There is generally an ebb and flow of activity, with stimulation and affective experience alternating with time for reflection, conceptualization, and objectivity. Students should have affective experiences with community contacts and not just with patients. The setting must also provide opportunities for experiencing different types of people, including lay, professional, and paraprofessional individuals. The clinical space and teaching space must be in close proximity in order that the arrangements may be client- and trainee-centered rather than faculty-centered.

If certain lessons are built into the setting, faculty and trainees can be freer to concentrate on essential knowledge and skills which require direct instruction. If all training occurs in a protected, homogeneous psychiatric treatment environment, then the program has difficulty providing balance and subspecialty diversification—faculty and students tend to deal with community and homes in fantasy and intellectually and only with sick patients and professional colleagues affectively. Consistent with this thesis, psychiatrists who were trained in the latter tradition and settings tend to carry deep convictions regarding the psychiatrist as a clinician and to be skeptical—in fact to lack knowledge and skills in depth—regarding other types of psychiatric work. Some trainees lack natural talent for psychotherapeutic work just as others lack talent for research, writing, teaching, consultation, community work, or administration.

The challenge of the field is not to provide high-quality direct care by psychiatrists for all who would benefit from it—this is manifestly and statistically impossible. The challenge is to promote a good match between the resourcefulness of those highly talented and trained persons who become physicians and psychiatrists, the resourcefulness of other colleagues, and the mental health needs of the population. Clinical settings should be of a nature and variety to foster that match. Clinical settings and educational programs can thus provide flexible accommodations among individual fulfillment, organizational function, institutonal purpose, and societal needs.

Discussion

A number of themes from the residency training discussion continued in this session. The core experience or curriculum for residency training would appear to be determined very much by the setting in which it occurs. Thus, the discussion focused on the problems involved in the shift from training in the traditional university hospital to the community hospital and community mental health center, from an inpatient orientation to an ambulatory emphasis. In addition to redefining core training experiences and considering the various kinds of psychiatrists who may emerge after the core experiences discussed in previous chapters, new medical schools are reexamining the essential connections between educational program and clinical setting, particularly when they find themselves operating their programs in a setting other than their own. As the prospect of interdisciplinary and generic training approaches, they are attempting to find its parameters. The major subtopics discussed and major alternative points of view surrounding them are presented here.

Mutual Influence of Setting and Program

An educational program seems to become built into the existing clinical setting and inexorably shaped by it. This is a subtle

71

process which often includes rationalizing the educational program based on the clinical setting unwittingly or unwillingly inherited—that is, making the best of what one has. While this adaptation may, at times, be healthy, some correctives should be provided.

Only five or six years ago "educational language"—setting objectives and then making the methods consistent with them—was rare. We now try to think of the whole educational program and the total institutional clinical objectives together. It is surprising how many times program directors seem uncertain about the foundation and historical base of their institution, let alone its present political and economic base. Although pure training objectives must often bend to real constraints within which they work, one can also capitalize on the assets and unique structure of the setting or institution. Instead, we often find program directors trying to fit round pegs into square holes, for instance by describing a program in a major urban receiving hospital as if it were serving the population base of an upper-class suburb. Knowing one's institution, identifying and capitalizing on its potential is critical.

Perhaps the most crucial factor in achieving maximum utilization of the clinical setting which serves the educational program is defining a population base so that the goal-setting process begins at the level of the community being served and its unique qualities and needs. If a program finds a catchment area, or part of one, which can serve as a training and research laboratory and a reference group, the sum of the goals of the training program can become congruent. Once the high-priority needs of the people being served are looked at, the manpower and training resources to serve these needs can be considered.

Educational "Control"

There is a difference between control of services and control of education, although the clinical policy of the institution relates the two. There may be parallel program directors, university-appointed, and clinical service directors, hospital-appointed. Some educational programs are content to control only their own operations and can work alongside the clinical services, particularly if they are affiliated with a variety of services and can develop ways to share control, that is, a consortium of institutions. The educators' principal task is to determine which aspects of the various settings they need to control. There is a drastic difference between the approach medical educators take in teaching students and that of the private practitioner. The discrepancies require much faculty time to help the people appointed in community hospitals discover how to deliver a learning experience that is meaningful.

It appears that most faculty members in new medical schools have not participated in designing the primary teaching facilities. However, the majority feel they can make major decisions about where students and residents are taught within the available facilities. Thus some departments teach in clinical facilities which do not belong to them, and who shall control quality of service becomes an important issue. Direct control is defined as that exercised by a chief of services from the departmental faculty who has power to appoint attending staff of the hospital. On the other hand, a "no control" situation exists when departmental teaching occurs in a facility run by the attending staff, so that ways of collaboration without direct control must then be worked out.

Many new schools, lacking access to public funds and facilities, have to work in private, attending-staff community hospitals. Here they face an entirely different control issue. How do they get the kind of quality care they would like to demonstrate to students as the model? The educational program will usually have less control over clinical operations in these private hospitals than in public hospitals where services are less highly developed and need the medical school input.

The blending of educational and service considerations will probably require time—perhaps twenty years for the marriage of the medical school and the community hospital to be firm. This goal also requires departments within the medical school to closely coordinate their objectives so that they do not create wide gaps or conflicting directions within a community hospital. Perhaps one common bond would be the medical school's working out an HMO agreement, thereby involving all the clinical departments in a common mission.

Most new medical schools seem to be aware that university involvement in service delivery is not best demonstrated by a fight over control but by contributing to experimental delivery systems which also serve educational purposes. A consortium of services, involving the university as a major partner and bringing together public and private agencies into a network of comprehensive service delivery, is one example.

Changing Delivery Systems

Traditionally it has been felt that students need to see severely ill patients who demonstrate dramatic symptomatology and to continue observing them during the treatment period. This traditional view reflects the belief that medical students and residents are best plunged into a ward to deal with serious chronic psychotic groups of patients so that the impact of learning psychopathology is real and very dramatic. A protected environment used to be thought important for the beginning trainee. The inpatient unit gives a concentrated affective experience "forcing" responsibility, which might occur with a suicidal patient: the student must make a judgment about letting the patient go home, then wonder about his judgment, not immediately following through with a telephone call but waiting. Visiting here and there in the community may dilute and contaminate the student's attempt to learn how to observe the interaction between himself and the patient. It is not possible in an outpatient setting to replicate this kind of condensed visual image of the changes that rapidly take place in inpatients. Today, however, some of this traditional experience can be preserved in partial hospitalization programs oriented to a variety of therapies—group, family, and marriage, as well as individual.

Another view suggests the key to good training is the appropriate model of care. Ambulatory care should make up most of the student's training because this type of care is what he will actually give in practice. Most physicians spend 90 percent of their time working with ambulatory patients rather than inpatients, so it does not make sense to do most of their training in an inpatient setting.

Some feel we should even go beyond thinking of psychiatric ambulatory settings, since the bulk of the ill in the country are not in mental health facilities but in general medical care settings. But most residents have little opportunity to do consultative liaison work in these settings. It has been found that roughly 25 percent of residency programs actually devote a significant amount of time to consultation liaison efforts. Integration with other medical disciplines is crucial, and the budding child psychiatrist should work with pediatrics, as an example.

General Principles

Much current thinking suggests that the particular sequence of training is less important than keeping in mind basic principles—early in his training a trainee needs a good deal of structure and supervision, which should decrease as his training progresses. One reason residents have been started on inpatient services is that there they encounter a very tight structure with close supervision. If a resident is immediately placed in a community or an outpatient setting, in which decision-making is much more difficult than it is in a hospital, where he has a good deal of help nearby, the setting must provide extra supervision and support.

Individual, intensive supervision, the most potent and effective teaching method psychiatry has, is the common denominator in any setting. However, by itself the method lacks the patient in context. Although the supervisor may bring a great deal of conceptual clarity to the student's description of his work with the patient, their interaction remains at an intellectual, cognitive level. Therefore, it is important that the student have an experience in the community, an experience that comes from direct contact in homes and on the street in order to develop his own clinical skills. This approach is called direct-action learning and is best done when the teacher is involved in doing the same thing the student is doing, is on the team with him, and is not just receiving material from the student.

Interdisciplinary Training

The crisis intervention centers now spawning around the country reveal how problems redefine the roles of people working on them. These services operate by walk-in or by telephone inquiry, and patients often do not know the particular mental health discipline of the person responding to them. All they know is that they are seeing crisis intervention workers. Frequently encountered problems have to do with drugs, alcoholism, abortion, psychosis, the need for money to buy food, placing aged people, problems of depression, homosexuality, sexual dysfunction, marital conflict, and child abuse. These are the subjects of modern psychiatric practice, and the student responding to them becomes the focus in mobilizing the care. This may be the psychiatric service model of the future and requires training much broader than that traditionally provided.

The country is moving toward a comprehensive health delivery system for all people, and within it the role for mental health may be changed. In mental health delivery—individual, family, and group therapies, crisis intervention, consultation, and education —there is a commonality which has no unique professional badge among the various mental health professions.

In many minority communities the best-trained professionals do not necessarily have the knowledge, the skill, the aptitude, the language and communication, and the traditions to understand the needs of the people living there. Community desire for control or sharing of power presses this issue even further, giving rise to the new careerists in mental health who often can respond to those particular needs and tasks that traditional professionals cannot or will not fulfill. With common functions already bridging the professional and paraprofessional disciplines, there may be an advantage in giving *all* people who will work together in a service delivery system of the future some experience learning together. The perspectives of the mental health disciplines and of new careerists must be brought together in planning and developing training programs.

Thus far the concept of interdisciplinary training has often been applied in a very naive way—simply placing people from nursing, social work, and medicine in the same room and lecturing to them simultaneously. This approach not only achieves little or nothing but may be a negative experience since it may arouse competitiveness among students rather than cooperation. The alternative appears to be to create experiences in which students work collaboratively in real settings, with the teachers who are serving as models illustrating how collaborative care works and what team involvement is all about.

Part Four

Planning and Evaluation of Training

Some new terms are appearing in professional education, even though they have long been known to educators. In the health professions, especially mental health, such concepts as "instructional objectives," "assessments of success in achieving objectives," and "the mastery model of education" have begun to receive notice in the past five years. Where before we spoke in terms of courses, topics, clerkships, and examinations, we are now being asked to formulate behavioral objectives, to design assessment procedures and entry profiles to measure student performance on the basis of success in achieving the objectives, and to introduce flexibility into the length of time expected or required for achieving a degree. For those involved in medical and psychiatric education before the educationists entered the field, this change has required a rather painful rethinking of educational strategies and tactics, as well as the learning of a whole new vocabulary and method of designing programs.

The next two chapters are by psychiatrists who are also educationists, a new breed that seems to be increasing in numbers. Dr. Jason presents the philosophy and conceptual framework in which objectives and priorities for instruction in psychiatry are grounded.

Dr. Templeton describes the most recent work being done in evaluating medical student performance in psychiatry, an appropriate companion piece to one on instructional objectives. The discussion section makes clear that the need for this new approach is appreciated by all but that it creates a major problem for the educator, who must learn a new vocabulary and a new methodology; also a great deal of time is required to redesign programs in terms of such objectives. An illustrative set of Guidelines for Competency Objectives in the Training of Mental Health Professionals in the First Year is included.

7

Instructional Objectives
and Priorities

HILLIARD JASON

Let us imagine that you are responsible for designing an entirely new program of instruction in psychiatry for medical students and that your only constraint is time. Whatever amount of time you have is clearly less than would be required to have students learn all of psychiatry, whatever that is. If you don't have time for everything, how do you decide what to include and what to omit? How do you get all the different instructors to agree on these decisions? You certainly recognize that if they don't agree, whether knowingly or unknowingly, they may be working at cross-purposes, and you will be stuck with a sadly inefficient program. What part can or should students play in this decision-making? And how should the results of these decisions be formulated so that they can be communicated to others?

Should the program, for example, include the development of interviewing skills? If so, which ones, and to what level of proficiency? Should it include an understanding of the distinctions among character disorders, neuroses, and psychoses? Just the understanding of these distinctions or the capacity to actually make them with patients? Should the history of psychiatry be included? Why? How will students make use of what they learn in this area? And then, should the program be concerned about such nondisciplinary matters as the students' capacity to initiate their own learning, or evaluate their own capacities and limitations, or follow through on responsibilities? Aren't these competencies fundamentally important in an effective physician? If so, whose task is it to help assure that they are fostered and developed?

Offering an instructional program without first asking and answering the many questions which I have posed or implied is nearly equivalent to setting out on a long vacation trip without ever considering where you are intending to go or which places you want to see or skip along the way. Left to pure chance, or momentary impulse, or unexamined intuition, as is much of conventional instruction, the trip would run a high risk of missing some of the most attractive highlights, squandering precious time and resources on unnecessary or even undesirable experiences, and ending up somewhere you really didn't want to be.

Our fond hopes notwithstanding, educational programs, like unplanned travel, can have negative outcomes. The student who has experiences which reinforce or cause a distrust of the motivations of psychiatrists or who becomes convinced that helping patients with emotional difficulties is out of reach of anyone but psychiatrists has derived seriously negative consequences from his education. Any capacity such a student may have for responding correctly on information-oriented psychiatry exams is vitiated by the overriding long-range damaging effects of the negative attitudes he has developed.

There is simply no escape from or shortcut to defining the intentions of an instructional program. It is hard work, but it is unavoidable if quality is to be achieved. The following are some central questions faculty members ask, or should ask, about instructional objectives, and some guides to their answers.

Why are objectives needed? In every area of human endeavor, one's specific intentions must be formulated in advance if there is to be consistent likelihood of success. Whether traveling, undertaking a research project, providing medical care, or offering instruction, as Bob Mager has said, "if you are not sure where you are going, you may end up somewhere else." There is simply not enough time to try to do everything. Choices have to be made. Whenever some content is included in an instructional unit, other content is omitted. Whenever questions are asked on specific topics in an evaluation, other areas go unexamined. The only way to be sure that the instruction and evaluation do deal with the highest priority issues is to define in advance what the priorities in fact are. The important point is: we *always* have objectives, whether we have managed to make them explicit or not. The material we include and exclude in our instruction and examinations defines our objectives. The risk in not having overtly defined them first is that things we really care about may get omitted and things which are trivial or even inappropriate can be emphasized.

What is meant by "behavioral" objectives? It has become fashionable for instructors in the health professions to acknowledge that they must specify their objectives in behavioral terms. Unfortunately, the purpose and method of such specification are not always fully understood. Faculty need to appreciate that objectives are only meaningful when they describe *observable* and *measurable* performance, not abstract or hypothetical states of mind that one hopes the student might have achieved. An objective should describe an overt competency that is appropriate for a physician or a prior level of achievement which will enable the subsequent development of such competencies. A meaningful objective, for example, might be: "all students will be able to gather sufficient data from any patient they interview to effectively describe that patient's mental status." This describes or suggests a specific set of behaviors. An objective which states that "each student will appreciate the importance of the mental status exam" is not meaningful. No behavior is suggested, and as a consequence the fulfillment of this objective is neither observable nor measurable. The question faculty members must ask themselves is, "How will I know that a student *appreciates* the importance of the mental status exam?" Our concern, as instructors, is with the behavior toward which such an appreciation will lead: the observable act of actually collecting and recording mental status data on all patients encountered, whether or not the student is being examined or is on a psychiatry service.

What is meant by "terminal" and "enabling" objectives?
The process of setting priorities and writing objectives forces confrontation with some of the basic questions in instructional program design. Those specific objectives that actually get written are merely expressions of the intentions or purposes of the overall instructional effort. In medical school, the intent is to produce general physicians, at a modest level of competence. A description of their intended characteristics, of those tasks they are to be able to perform, the skills they can demonstrate, the steps they can take in problem-solving, and so on would be a set of terminal objectives for the medical school's overall program. One such objective might be the expectation regarding the mental status examination mentioned earlier. Most terminal objectives, including this one, are sufficiently complex so that they cannot be fully achieved in a single instructional step. Instead, a sequential learning experience is, or should be, devised which provides a set of interrelated steps which build on each other. Among the necessary steps for achieving the objective of gathering data for an effective mental status exam are: the capacity to conduct a systematic interview: an understanding of the concepts of abstract and concrete thinking; and the ability to generate questions which tap the resources of short-term and long-term memory. Each of these is an enabling objective in the realization of the desired terminal objective. As is sometimes true with other enabling objectives, the first of these three is itself a terminal objective in a medical school curriculum. Problems arise when items that are merely enabling objectives begin to be treated as though they were terminal objectives, in and of themselves. This misrepresentation occurs frequently with regard to the content of the preclinical sciences, but it is also a trap into which we can fall in fashioning parts of a psychiatric curriculum. Clearly, we have formulated a behavioral objective when we have stated that "students will be able to describe and interrelate the concepts of progression, fixation, and regression in human development." That this statement describes a set of behaviors is not enough. We must be cautious not to lose sight of the fact that this is an enabling, not a terminal objective. It is meant to facilitate the student's comprehension of mechanisms which are operative in real patients, with real problems. If his teachers lose sight of this interrelationship, and the student,

as a consequence, is led to believe that his description of these three concepts is an end in itself, there is a serious risk that he will reject these concepts as just so much more esoterica, of peculiar interest to the psychiatrist but irrelevant to other physicians. The terminal objective(s) toward which this enabling objective points must have been clearly forumlated in advance and must be in the forefront of the thinking of both teacher and student as they deal with this material, if the negative consequences are to be avoided.

Can objectives really be written for the complex and subtle issues that characterize psychiatry? Objectives can be written more easily in some areas than in others. The assertion can be made, however, that objectives can, and indeed must, be specified for any area taught. But for some complex subjects it is difficult or unreasonable to try to specify all the possible performances which are meant to derive from instruction. It is more reasonable under such circumstances to focus on specifying priorities among groups of objectives and have the specific details emerge in the course of instruction itself. To illustrate: in developing objectives for the doctor-patient relationship, it may be satisfactory to specify that students will, for example, be helped to develop a consistent pattern of avoiding any remarks or behavior which may be censoring or constraining to the patient. A few illustrations would then help make the point, but it would not be reasonable to try and develop the compendium necessary to define every possible constraining or censoring behavior or, the reverse, all possible facilitating behaviors.

How specific and detailed must written objectives be? It is actually best to begin at quite a general level, because here the issue of priorities can best be confronted. For example, in planning objectives for psychiatry, the first step is finding answers to the difficult question: "What are the highest priority intentions of the overall instructional program?" It seems to me that among them might be such goals as assuring that all students are attuned to the affective components of whatever problems their patients have; capable of, and committed to, managing minor emotional disorders in their patients; able to recognize serious emotional disorders for which psychiatric consultation is indicated; able to establish the kind of empathic, trust-based relationship with their patients that makes the foregoing possible. Given these sorts of general goals, plus any others the faculty agree deserve consideration, all subsequent goals and specific objectives must be evaluated in terms of their support for, or risk of detraction from, these goals. Clearly, specific objectives can only be written after these priority decisions have been made.

What are some useful strategies for beginning to identify the topics and areas for which objectives should be written? Instructors should understand that whether or not they have ever even thought about instructional objectives they do, in fact, have objectives which have been in operation as long as they have had an instructional program. Their objectives have been specified, indirectly, through the topics selected for coverage in class, the reading assignments, and the examinations or other evaluation devices used. It is often helpful to review past instruction and evaluation procedures to identify or derive their implicit objectives. Sometimes this review becomes an effective first step in further elaborating and refining the group's objectives, and sometimes it becomes a basis for departure, when the instructor recognizes that excessive attention had inadvertently been given to objectives which, on reflection, have lower priority than intended, or even negative, value. Additional steps can be sitting in on and observing classes in process; talking with students about their perceptions of the objectives that are being achieved and their views on those that should be achieved; and analyzing the actual task demands faced by those who are now in medical practice. All the data gathered through these various devices, however, must be interpreted and used against the perspective of the best judgment of the wisest and most highly informed individuals that can be gathered, who must try to predict the nature of the demands which physicians will encounter in the future. Merely defining objectives according to what is now taught, or according to what physicians now do, is to guarantee early obsolescence.

Are different objectives needed for different levels (years or phases) of the school's program? Initially, every teaching unit within a school should formulate its objectives in terms of only one level: the competencies required for graduation from that school. Ultimately, those must be the criteria against which all instructional decisions are measured. Once these objectives have been formulated, two other types of decisions can be made. First, are there lower levels of performance of the same competencies that will be expected at earlier stages in the program? (Might the goals of interviewing competency, for example, be applicable at several earlier stages in the program, but at lower levels of proficiency?) And second, are other objectives needed to serve as enabling objectives for achieving the ones specified? (As discussed earlier, are there some competencies, such as knowing various modes of psychological adaptation that occur during development, which are not part of the school's terminal objectives but which must be specified for earlier phases because they facilitate or permit the realization of one or more terminal objectives?) In either of these two cases, the program becomes defined in terms of a rational, interrelated sequence, so that it is a continuum rather than a collection of discrete, nonrelated experiences.

Are objectives to be written for each separate course? At first, departments should conceptualize their objectives independently of their current course offerings. The need is to define objectives in terms of the competencies expected of graduates. Only secondarily should attention be given to how these abilities will be developed. The central point is that there should be multiple avenues for fulfilling these objectives, including the recognition that some students will already have achieved these competencies as a consequence of prior experience and need not be required to engage in whatever instruction is offered. Even those students who do not yet possess the skills intended should have alternative methods for achieving these objectives, according to their different learning rates and learning styles. In fact, courses should be shaped, or reshaped, according to the objectives the department defines, rather than the reverse.

How can the quality and appropriateness of each objective be evaluated? Whenever possible, every objective in its final form should meet the following criteria: (1) Clarity. The statement should be sufficiently clear and communicative so that a person who is moderately familiar with the instructional area could independently describe in some detail the student performance which is expected, on the basis of reading the objective. Note: An objective may be sufficiently clear and appropriately written and yet not be fully communicative to a beginning student. It is often necessary to have some comprehension of the field in question (in other words, to have partially achieved the objective itself) before the intent of the objective is fully understood. (2) Assessability. The behavior(s) expected is (are) described with sufficient specificity, and adequate criteria are provided, so that there is no question about the possibility of, or approach to, evaluating student performance in this area. The minimal acceptable level of performance should be specified so there is no ambiguity about the requirements for satisfactory completion of a unit. (3) Relevance. Physicians from discipline areas other than the one formulating the objectives should agree to the appropriateness of each objective, in terms of its relevance to medicine and medical practice.

Will exams and other evaluation procedures have to be restricted to the areas covered in the list of objectives? In a word, yes. If there is anything a faculty member or group wishes to evaluate for which objectives have not yet been written, then objectives should be written in that area. It is important for faculty to understand that the objectives themselves should serve as a blueprint in guiding the development of all evaluation procedures.

Doesn't the approach of defining objectives in terms of "minimal acceptable performance" lead to mediocrity? It is essential to understand that there is no necessary relationship between (1) specifying that level of performance which is the *minimum* acceptable and (2) being willing to accept a minimal (low) level of performance. That level which is to be acceptable could, in fact, be defined as being of superior quality. This issue is at the heart of the evolution of a mastery-based curriculum. The difference is between defining in advance how well one's graduates will perform in each required area and the more characteristic approach of making ad hoc decisions each year, on the basis of how well the average student happens to perform. In conventional programs, without prior specification of the minimum acceptable level, there is a real risk that the standard will be set by the majority, which in a given year may happen to be mediocre.

Aren't objectives constricting and restraining? The fairly common posture of expecting objectives to be highly detailed has led to the misunderstanding that only those things which are highly specifiable, in performance terms, are definable as objectives. The tendency, as a consequence, is to assume that only trivial learning can be specified as behavioral objectives. In point of fact, any expectation a faculty member may have can be formulated as an objective, including such expectations as having students identify areas of personal interest beyond those specified in the defined objectives, which will then be pursued to some identified level of competence. In other words, evidence of independent initiative and creativity, and other similarly complex performance, can be required by suitably written objectives.

There are other questions that should be asked, and answered, about objectives, but they are probably subissues or refinements of those I have posed. If faculty members in a department can become committed to the principles embedded in the responses I discussed, they will be in an effective position to sort out most additional problems that might arise in formulating objectives.

While the principles outlined or implied in this chapter are necessary as a basis for setting instructional objectives, they are of no value unless program priorities have been appropriately defined in the first place. Carefully refining objectives which merely elaborate unreasonable or irrelevant goals is a waste of everyone's time; in fact, this activity may be dangerous if it brings an air of systematization and the trappings of quality to a program that really needs to be changed or abandoned.

Clearly, the turning point in the quality of instructional design is the quality and appropriateness of those goals that are defined as being top priority. While it is important to help educate all faculty members to recognize the importance of this issue, it is vital that the most able thinking that can be mobilized be brought to bear on the actual process of priority-setting. The necessary wisdom and vision, in addition to competence in instructional design, are rare commodities which must be pursued and cultivated if all the other program development efforts are to be worth the trouble.

Evaluating Student Performance

BRYCE TEMPLETON

≋≋≋≋≋≋≋≋≋≋≋≋≋≋≋≋≋≋≋≋≋≋≋≋≋≋≋≋

*F*or centuries, Western universities have used essay examinations as a major method of assessing student performance. Although they are still widely used, ample evidence documents their serious limitations: problems related to sampling, the absence of norms, the halo effect of grammar and spelling, and especially the lack of test reliability (Charvat and others, 1968). This concept of reliability has played an important role in the development of the testing field. The term *reliability* refers to the degree to which a test or other evaluation technique can be relied upon to provide consistent and reproducible results. The lack of reliability of essay examinations can be demonstrated by comparing the scores assigned to a single set of papers by two or more instructors or by comparing an initial set of scores assigned by one instructor with a second set of scores assigned by the same instructor reviewing the same group of papers after a brief interval of time.

Multiple-Choice Tests

The National Board of Medical Examiners made extensive use of the essay method until the early 1950s. At that time the multiple-choice technology began to exert its influence on students and physicians qualifying for license or specialty board certification; this new evaluation technique had entered medical education through a liaison between the National Board and representatives of a new specialty within the field of education, namely, the field of testing and measurement (Hubbard, 1971; Stokes, 1967; Womack, 1965). In spite of the progessive growth of medical school programs in psychiatry throughout the 1940s and 1950s, psychiatry missed out on participation in the essay era (because there were no separate psychiatry exams then) as far as the National Board was concerned. Considering the limited merits of essay examinations, this was no great loss. But to the extent that this omission reflected an unfamiliarity with and disinterest in examination technology, it might have served as a warning to psychiatric educators that they should familiarize themselves with a field which would continue to exert a major influence on their educational programs for decades to come.

The multiple-choice methodology provided solutions to many of the problems associated with essay examinations; in particular, it vastly improved the sampling of subject matter and provided a highly reliable measuring device. The advent of machine scoring and the availability of computer data processing have not only saved us from hours of drudgery but have also provided valuable information about the usefulness of individual test items (Charvat and others, 1968; Jason, 1966). However, this feedback has helped to dispell any uncertainty about the need for careful preparation of examination materials. Considerable time is required for a group of colleagues to write and then jointly review one another's materials. This process is essential in order to eliminate ambiguous phrasing, to assure broadly based relevance, to maintain an appropriate level of difficulty, and to maximize the likelihood that answers to individual test items reflect more than one individual's whimsical bias.

I have some reservations about the advisability of individual medical schools undertaking construction of multiple-choice examinations. It is time-consuming and costly, and there are other aspects of evaluating student performance which should command higher priority on faculty time. If a medical school faculty feels strongly that it should develop its own multiple-choice examinations in psychiatry and behavioral sciences, I urge that it do the following. First, it should contact a college of education in a nearby university to purchase some consulting services to assist in designing the examination, writing individual items, and working out arrangements for machine scoring and simple statistical analysis describing the performance of individual test items. Second, the faculty should make inquiries among other medical schools to see whether a cooperative effort can be developed to distribute the work load and to share the finished product. At the present time, there is a tremendous need for a nationally available pool of psychiatry test items that local faculties might draw on to provide both students and faculty with interim feedback about one another's progress. The National Board has, of course, developed a sizable pool of test items. However, because our licensure examinations rely on a sampling technique, our pool of test items is still too small to make public without risking the likelihood that these test items would become a textbook which students would inappropriately use to the exclusion of other important study materials.

Testing with Films

One important modification of conventional multiple-choice testing involves the use of these test items in conjunction with sound film or videotape presentations of real or simulated interviews. Several groups have used this approach to assess observational skills and the ability to understand interview material.

Our experiences at the National Board using the combination of filmed material and multiple-choice questions finally led to our abandoning this technique. Since the early 1960s, test committee members representing the disciplines of internal medicine, obstetrics, pediatrics, and surgery had been producing films for our Part III examination (given during the latter part of internship), designed primarily to assess observational skills and knowledge of physical examination findings (Levit, 1967). We used color film to provide greater flexibility in demonstrating physical examination findings and made sufficient copies for simultaneous administration in eighty to ninety examination centers. Producing and duplicating color films was an expensive operation. In addition, the item analysis and indices of reliability of this section of the examination did not meet the standards to which we had become accustomed with conventional multiple-choice material. Specifically, many of the test items were too easy or too difficult and failed to discriminate between a more able group and a less able group.

Nevertheless, in 1969 we began to develop some examination films concerned with interviewing skills. We decided that we would again have to use color film or else run the risk of giving candidates obvious cues to pay special attention to psychological factors during black and white film presentations. A review of the item analysis data for individual test items together with a determination of over-all reliability for this section of the examination revealed that we had been unsuccessful in appreciably improving on the marginal performance noted before. After vigorous discussions among the staff and test committee, we abandoned the use of filmed material.

Enelow has developed a somewhat different technique which also combines the use of multiple-choice test items with film presentations, but it is designed to focus on the physician's verbal interventions. He used this technique to compare the effects of a programmed film series on interviewing with the effects of several other instructional methods (Enelow, 1970). His filmed interviews stop periodically at certain nodal points and the examinee is requested to select the best of three options indicating how he thinks the doctor should respond at each of these points. The choices of responses include asking open-ended questions, using confrontation, asking direct questions, maintaining silence, providing advice, and so on.

As one becomes increasingly familiar with examinations, a question naturally arises: are these multiple-choice tests evaluating students in those areas that really count? This question refers to that property of an examination known as validity. The term *validity* is defined as the extent to which an examination actually measures what it purports to measure. It seems reasonable to assume that a physician cannot provide adequate care for his patients without a substantial amount of medical knowledge; yet attempts to assess the validity of multiple-choice examinations by determining the degree of correlation between performance on the examinations and estimates of the quality of day-to-day care subsequently provided by the same physician have been disappointing (Colmore, 1966; Gonnella, 1970; Price and others, 1964). Indeed, one study comparing the performance of medical students on an examination concerning knowledge of interviewing techniques with ratings of observed interviewing behavior demonstrated a significantly negative correlation (Ware and others, 1971). Although some argue that the measures of the quality of day-to-day physician performance are not sufficiently reliable, the results of each of these studies have been consistently in the same direction.

In my opinion, evaluating a physician's knowledge still represents an important aspect of assessing his clinical competence, but, frankly, I am pessimistic that written examinations will provide us with an effective means of assessing interpersonal skills. Nor will multiple-choice examinations provide the quality control necessary to assure that the physician's knowledge is applied in his day-to-day performance.

Human Simulations

Most of the detailed outlines specifying the elements constituting physician competence include certain interpersonal skills such as information-gathering interviewing and simple psychotherapeutic maneuvers. It is unfortunate, therefore, that written examinations, which have played such an important role in evaluating medical students and physicians, do such a poor job of assessing these behaviors.

In the past, a variety of groups have attempted to test interpersonal skills by directly observing the examinee with an actual patient. Even though careful preparation of examiners and use of rating scales can significantly improve the reliability of an examiner's rating of an interview, variations in the patients and the challenge they pose for the examinee seriously restrict the reliability of this technique. For example, it is meaningless to compare, for examination purposes, the performance of one student who is forced to dig for information from a seventy-year-old man with significant loss of recent memory with that of a second student whose patient responds to his initial question with an uninterrupted account of most of the important history findings related to the patient's present illness (Scott, 1970).

The development of the simulated patient may represent a

milestone in the history of assessing the interpersonal aspects of physician competence (Barrows, 1964). Paid actors (or occasionally the examiners themselves) are programmed to simulate a specific patient with a specific illness, history, personality, and life style. A number of actors can simulate the same patient, and a large number of examinees can, in effect, interview the same patient (Barrows, 1971; Levine, 1968). The use of simulated patients avoids the tremendous variation in patient characteristics inevitably associated with the use of actual patients and thereby increases the reliability of the assessment.

The work of Helfer, Hess, and Jason, using simulated patients for both educational and evaluative purposes, is providing valuable insights into this approach. For example, Helfer's discovery of a decline in psychosocial data-gathering skills during the first two years of medical school is a startling documentation of behavior which many have suspected for some time (Helfer, 1970; Helfer and Hess, 1970). The work of these investigators offers hope that the use of human simulated patients will provide a reasonably reliable, valid, and economically feasible method of episodic assessment of interpersonal skills.

Unfortunately, our existing medical licensing and specialty board certifying procedures do not require physicians to demonstate competence in interpersonal skills. This deficit gives the budding physician an important message: although a certain fund of medical knowledge is an essential attribute of the practicing physician, interpersonal skills are too ill-defined, too ambiguous, or of insufficient importance for him to be concerned about during preparations for certifying examinations. Psychiatric departments might well consider using simulated patients as a way to evaluate the competence of medical students. Efforts of individual medical schools to assess interpersonal skills will hold special importance until the day when national licensing programs adopt some equally effective method.

Quality Control Audits

Academic psychiatrists who have carried on liaison teaching activities in the wards and clinics administered by other clinical departments are probably all too familiar with the difficulties associated with getting physicians-in-training to apply in these other clinical settings the knowledge and skills supposedly learned during their formal training in psychiatry. When this ineptness is observed in house-officer graduates from other medical schools, it is easy to dismiss the problem as the unfortunate result of a weak department in that other school. However, one cannot so easily rationalize the failure to apply elementary psychiatric knowledge on the part of able students who have rotated successfully through one's own clinical clerkship in psychiatry.

Two techniques offer great promise in dealing with this impairment in the transfer of learning: audits of medical record entries and audits of audio-taped student-patient interactions. The medical chart audit apparently originated from the establishment of tissue committees by surgeons who wished to provide an element of quality control over one another's operating room activities. In recent years several groups have devised audits of different types to assess the appropriateness of hospital bed utilization, to describe patient care practices, to estimate the quality of hospital and office care provided by individual physicians, and to assess the impact of continuing education programs (Beaumont and others, 1967; Donabedian, 1966; Lembcke, 1967; Morehead, 1967). Recently, Weed (1969) has effectively called attention to the need for careful thought concerning the organization of what goes into the patient's record (for example, his concept of the problem-oriented record) and the educational importance attached to students' careful review of chart entries. The results of several chart audit studies suggest that an awareness by the physician that certain aspects of his chart entries are being systematically reviewed is often associated with improvement in that aspect of patient care (Williamson, 1967).

Psychiatrists and other medical educators have been reviewing medical records for years. How, then, does a chart audit differ from this traditional supervisory activity? The development of a chart audit (1) requires some collaborative work by a hospital staff or faculty to determine which elements in a chart should be reviewed; (2) requires quantification of the extent to which the medical record entries meet or surpass certain minimum standards; (3) usually involves mechanizing the audit procedure so that the routine abstracting can be performed economically by trained nonphysician auditors; (4) requires randomizing the selection of charts which will actually be audited; and most importantly (5) should involve a review of a sample of all of a student's chart entries, not just those entries concerning his psychiatric patients.

In a study by the author, an eighty-seven-item chart audit was used to review the performance of twenty-one medical students in a medical outpatient clinic. The eighty-seven items were divided into six categories: (1) the patient's relationship to important people in his life, such as mother, father, and spouse; (2) important life events, such as education, employment, and illness; (3) special problems, such as difficulty handling aggression, neurotic symptoms, difficulties with sexual adjustment, and sleep disturbances; (4) a mental status examination, including estimates of mood, memory, and intelligence; (5) psychosocial diagnoses, such as standard psychiatric diagnostic terms, certain medical diagnoses with commonly recognized psychological implications (such as essential hypertension), and social problems; and (6) plans involving further psychiatric study or treatment, such as psychological testing, referral to social service, use of psychotropic agents, or psychotherapy.

The audit of these student-patient encounters demonstrated a narrow range of student performance with relatively little psychosocial data being elicited. Students reported information about alcohol, drug abuse, anxiety, and sleep disturbances; but they rarely obtained information concerning interpersonal relationships, important changes in patients' lives, or problems dealing with sex, aggression, and interracial conflict. They rarely explored temporal relationships between psychological disequilibrium and illness onset, and only infrequently gave written indication of any plan to follow up the few psychiatric problems which were identified.

A similar audit applied to tape recordings of the same student-patient encounters demonstrated that the chart closely reflected that which transpired during the course of the interview and physical examination, insofar as the gathering of information from the patient and the identification of medical and psychological problems were concerned. Informal observations of some of the same medical students interviewing patients in the psychiatric outpatient clinic indicated that they dealt with patients identified as having psychiatric problems in a very different manner in terms of the type of psychosocial information obtained, the types of problems identified, and willingness to follow through in attempting to alleviate the patient's problems.

The audit procedure provides the means of assessing certain student attitudes, including his willingness to apply his psychiatric knowledge and skills in all clinical settings. In addition, the process of auditing a sample of all of a student's chart entries tells the student that a psychiatry department regards the body of knowledge and skills which he studied during his brief psychiatric clerkship as essential in meeting the minimum standards for acceptable patient care.

Even though chart entries may accurately reflect the information obtained from patients by medical students, there are a number of interviewing and psychotherapeutic behaviors whose day-to-day performance may require a more direct method of quality control: for example, the student's ability to use a balance of open-ended versus direct questions, the ability to follow up on leads, and the ability to use silence. Occasional direct observation of specific interviews, after the initial skills are learned, runs the risk that behavior during a specially observed encounter may differ substantially from habitual behavior with patients. In addition, any quality control procedure involving direct observation would be exceedingly costly in terms of faculty time.

The development of tape recorders revolutionized the supervision of interviewing and psychotherapeutic skills of medical students and residents. Now, with the availability of relatively inexpensive cassette recorders, faculty and students have an opportunity to use recorded material in a much more systematic fashion. The sharing of one cassette recorder by two students, each of whom records all his patient contacts on alternate weeks, could provide the faculty with an especially valuable tool for evaluating the application of interviewing and psychotherapeutic skills in a wide variety of clinical settings. Supervision conducted on a group basis, the monitoring of only small segments of the recorded material, the reuse of the cassette tapes, and the training of students or other nonphysician educational assistants to provide constructive critiques of the recorded sessions would all help to make this arrangement economically feasible.

Computer Simulations

In the past two decades computers have gained increasing recognition as instructional devices. With the availability of typewriter keyboard or touch-sensitive, cathode-ray tube input and teletypewriter or cathode-ray tube display output, computers can be programmed to simulate many clinical problems. These simulations permit a medical student or resident to learn to deal effectively with a variety of situations before having to confront them in real life (Colby, 1966; Harless, 1971). Computer simulations will also permit the student's instructors to examine his ability to match the recommended method of handling various clinical problems. In all likelihood, computer simulations will permit assessment of behavior which is relevant to departmental objectives but which may be difficult to assess with other evaluative methods: for instance, willingness to obtain mental status information, or the selection of noncued options, such as requesting medical records from another hospital or talking with a member of the patient's family to obtain additional history.

One may argue that a computer simulation is too artificial, that it omits nonverbal communication, and that the lexical exchange lacks the natural flow of a real interview. Nevertheless, I predict that computer simulations will play a significant role in the future evaluation of physician competence, and I urge psychiatrists to become actively involved in designing these patient simulations. I hope that if faculty members have not already done so they will take advantage of computer simulation demonstrations which periodically appear at national conventions.

Summary

Multiple-choice examinations will probably continue to serve a useful role in assessing a young physician's knowledge of medicine. However, it seems unlikely that multiple-choice techniques will be able to examine interviewing or other interpersonal skills. At the moment, the use of human simulators offers the most promise in this area. In addition, we need to place a high priority on developing quality control measures, which, in turn, will help students learn to apply their psychiatric knowledge and skills in all clinical settings. Systematic audits of student chart entries and audio-tape interactions with patients should effectively aid students' translation of essential knowledge into effective day-to-day patient care. Finally, developments in computer simulation of clinical problems as a method of evaluating medical competence will require active input from psychiatrists in order to make this technique capable of evaluating and reinforcing many of the educational objectives of psychiatric educational programs.

Discussion

The difficulty in designing instructional objectives and developing assessments for examining systems was discussed. The question was raised about whether or not medical schools could pool their work and organize to create a document of instructional objectives useful to all. The problem seems to be that this pooling requires a considerable investment of time, and what may be applicable in one setting may not in another. Jason pointed out that it is harder to train people to think in terms of instructional objectives than it is to actually formulate them, once the appropriate philosophy has been accepted.

A second issue discussed was the need for an entry profile on each student before undertaking to provide instructional objectives appropriate to each one. Experiments at Michigan State University in creating such entry profiles were described by Jason. Once these profiles have been devised, the next problem will be periodic evaluations and the necessity to allow for a variety of entry points, as well as entry assessments for the various phases of a given curriculum, in order to have an orderly progression for the students as they learn more and are capable of undertaking increasingly complex tasks.

The need for a series of evaluations means that new ways of

99

assessing student behavior must be developed, particularly premedical training. What is required is a relevant approach to predicting the suitability of a given student for entering medicine. Such measures would be part of a premedical educational and evaluative experience.

Can residents be used to evaluate students as well as to teach them? It was agreed that both residents and students could be educated to teach and evaluate other students. A rich potential resource of instructional manpower in these days of short dollars is the students themselves.

Templeton described some interesting experiments in developing interrater reliability by a group that was assessing day-to-day student performance. They worked closely together, agreed on the definitions of the variables to be assessed, and compared data at regular intervals, eventually achieving a reliability of around .80.

In evaluating students for entrance, the focus on science grades and grade-point averages should be replaced by emphasis on those competencies that are part of medicine—such as the ability to assemble, modify, and reject facts, to relate to people, to take responsibility for one's own learning, and to be honest and responsible.

Several students spoke and emphasized the following points: Premedical studies do not seem to be very relevant to what goes on in a medical education. There is an overemphasis on science in premedical education and on basic science in medical education. Many people with appropriate personal characteristics for medical practice but who do not have a sufficiently high grade-point average fail to be accepted to medical school. There seemed to be unanimity among the students and residents attending the conference.

Jason questioned whether or not some schools are now recruiting disadvantaged students more for the sake of public appearance than for service to the individual being recruited. He felt that many such students who have been recruited have been treated irresponsibly. Another discussant felt that medical school administrators have been unwilling to agree to the degree of flexibility that is really needed to educate disadvantaged students in a medical school.

One way to provide the necessary flexibility is by applying the mastery model, which is based on defining the competencies, skills, and knowledge that the education planners of a particular school prescribe for graduates. These goals are formulated as instructional objectives. Due consideration is given to the fact that different people have different rates of learning, so that each student may take as long as he might need, within reason, to achieve these objectives. This program would have an entry evaluation, modular packages so that students can progress according to individual design, and periodic evaluation along the way for identifying deficiencies. Part of such a flexible curriculum would also be an examination of the qualifications necessary to practice medicine in different settings, so that students can prepare for the settings in which they intend to practice.

The lack of flexibility of the university may be a major constraint in providing variable-length training programs. A related problem is the fact that the National Board of Medical Examiners' standards were not set in the mastery-model concept, and the failure rates have been based on a group going through a course in standardized period of time. The scores of students trained in the mastery model will inaccurately reflect their knowledge and skills until NBME standards incorporate this model.

To illustrate the development of guidelines for competency objectives we include a set of such guidelines for the training of mental health professionals in the first year which were developed by the Department of Psychiatry of Pacific Medical Center. Included are: diagnostic knowledge and skills; interview skills; treatment knowledge and skills; psychological and social factors; psychiatry an the law; personal and professional growth; psychotherapy; and social and community psychiatry. Under each of these general headings, specific objectives are listed. For each objective, the method of assessing that objective and the setting in which that skill is taught are listed. A key to the teaching settings and clinical areas precedes the list of guidelines for competency objectives.

Key to Teaching Settings

1. Interviewing Seminar
2. Consultation Seminar
3. Psychotherapy Seminar
4. Somatic Therapy Seminar

5. Social and Community Psychiatry Seminar
6. Chairman's Seminar
7. Weekly Grand Rounds
8. Group Supervision and Development Seminar
9. Literature Seminar
10. Personality Development Seminar
11. Psychotherapy Supervision

Key to Clinical Areas

a. Inpatient Management
b. Outpatient Management
c. Day Treatment Center Patient Management
d. Intake Teams
e. Group Training
f. 3/4-Way Hospitalization
g. Charila (a residential treatment center for adolescent girls)
h. Other Community Agencies

Diagnostic Knowledge and Skills

Objective 1. The mental health professional differentiates between discrete behaviors and levels of inference about behaviors.

Assessment: orientation—observation of interviews; periodic assessment; patient work-ups.

Teaching settings and clinical areas: 1, 3, 7; a–e.

Objective 2. The mental health professional identifies the following patient characteristics as relevant to his diagnostic formulation: (A) physical appearance; (B) attire; (C) hygiene; (D) psychomotor reactions (e.g., agitation, retardation); (E) physiological reactions (such as blushing, sweating, gross changes in respiration rates); (F) cognitive reactions (e.g., intellect, though progression); (G) emotional reactions (such as affective reactions—anger, weeping, withdrawal, inappropriate laughter).

Assessment: orientation—observation of interviews; periodic assessment; patient work-ups.

Teaching settings and clinical areas: 1, 2, 3, 7; a–e.

Objective 3. The mental health professional can recognize and describe the central features of the following major psychiatric diagnoses: schizophrenia; affective psychosis; organic brain syndrome; neurotic depression; hysterical neurosis; anxiety; phobic state; sociopathic; hysterical and compulsive personality; addictions; mental retardation; and sexual problems.

Assessment: orientation—observation of interviews; periodic assessment; patient work-ups.

Teaching settings and clinical areas: 1, 2, 3, 7; a–e.

Objective 4. The mental health professional differentiates between his diagnostic impression and other likely diagnostic possibilities related to a given patient.

Assessment: orientation—observation of interviews; periodic assessment; patient work-ups.

Teaching settings and clinical areas: 1, 2, 3, 7; a–e.

Objective 5. The mental health professional can (A) describe the behaviors observed in a family group; (B) infer the family process from the observed behavior; (C) assess family functioning and estimate degree of psychopathology.

Assessment: case presentation; supervisor assessment; tutor assessment; patient management.

Teaching settings and clinical areas: 2, 7, 9, 10; a–h.

Objective 6. The mental health professional can (A) describe the behaviors observed in a group setting; (B) use his observations to understand the process of the group.

Assessment: group psychotherapy supervision; tutor assessment.

Teaching settings and clinical areas: 5, 8; a–h.

Interview Skills

Objective 1. The mental health professional demonstrates (A) the ability to listen to a patient; (B) the ability to help patients with problems in the psychological and psychiatric area; (C) the ability to establish and maintain a working relationship with a patient.

Assessment: orientation evaluation; periodic assessment; supervision; case conference presentations.

Teaching settings and clinical areas: 1, 2, 3, 11; a–d.

Objective 2. The mental health professional describes verbal and nonverbal cues in himself. *Objective 2(a)*. The mental health professional recognizes his own emotional needs as they are elicited in the interview.

Assessment: supervisor evaluation; periodic review; orientation evaluation.

Teaching settings and clinical areas: 1, 11; a–d.

Objective 3. The mental health professional does not permit his own emotional needs to interfere with his responding appropriately to the patient's emotional and physical needs. *Objective 3(a)*. The mental health professional is aware of the significance of his own personal background in his reactions to a patient's problem.

Assessment: supervisor evaluation; periodic review; orientation evaluation.

Teaching settings and clinical areas: 1, 11; a–d.

Objective 4. The mental health professional is able to elicit data relating to previous objectives by means of the mental status, physical, neurological, and psychological examinations.

Assessment: case conferences; patient management skills; periodic review; tutor assessment.

Teaching settings and clinical areas: 1, 2, 7; a–d.

Objective 5. The mental health professional is aware of the significance of his reactions: (A) to failure of his treatment; (B) to the dying patient; (C) to the suicidal or depressed patient; (D) to the demanding (manipulative) patient; (E) to the psychotic patient; (F) to the hostile or explosive patient; (G) to the silent and withdrawn patient; (H) to staff needs and expectations of him.

Assessment: supervisor assessment; periodic review; tutor assessment.

Teaching settings and clinical areas: 8, 11; a–d.

Objective 6. The mental health professional, in discussing with his supervisor interviews with any patient, demonstrates that he is aware of the relative merits of his considering and employing alternative ways of responding to the person.

Assessment: Supervisor assessment; case conference presentation; periodic review.

Teaching settings and clinical areas: 1, 3; a–d.

Objective 7. In subsequent interviews, the mental health professional demonstrates his ability to make adjustments in his overt behavior as a result of feedback on his performance.

Assessment: supervisor assessment; tutor assessment.

Teaching settings and clinical areas: 8, 11; a–d.

Treatment Knowledge and Skills

Objective 1. The mental health professional can describe what approach he will take with the patient (attitude, manner, and strategy) and how it relates to his treatment aims.

Assessment: patient management; case conference presentation; supervisor assessment; tutor assessment.

Teaching settings and clinical areas: 2, 3, 4, 7, 11; a–e.

Objective 2. In a given case, the mental health professional can describe and demonstrate his ability to carry out crisis intervention strategies appropriate to that case.

Assessment: patient management; intake team assessment.

Teaching settings and clinical areas: 1, 2, 4, 5; b, c, g, h.

Objective 3. The mental health professional can describe criteria and dosage for use of common psychiatric medications (chlorpromazine, trifluoperozine thioridazine, fluphenazine amitriptyline, imipramine, diazepam, chlordiazepoxide, phenobarbital, meprobamate, lithium carbonate, benztropine, trihexyphenidyl, glutethimide, paraldehyde, secoebarbital, chloral hydrate, methyprylon, diphenhydramine, methyl phenidate, dextro amphetamine), their side and toxic effects.

Assessment: patient management; tutor assessment; intake team assessment.

Teaching settings and clinical areas: 4, 9; a, b, c, d.

Objective 3(a). The mental health professional can describe criteria for use of somatic treatments (ECT; lobotomy, and its modifications; insulin coma; and other organic therapies), their side and toxic effects.

Assessment: patient management; tutor assessment; intake team assessment.

Teaching settings and clinical areas: 4; a, b, c, d.

Objective 4. On the basis of the diagnosis, the mental health profes-

sional knows the indications for: (A) special tests and examinations
(such as laboratory tests, EEG, LP, skull films, psychometrics,
Rorschach, Thematic Apperception Test, Bender-Gestalt, MMPI,
WAIS, WISC); (B) appropriate consultations and/or referral.

Assessment: patient management; case conference presentation; intake team assessment.

Teaching settings and clinical areas: 7, 9; a, b, c, d.

Objective 5. The mental health professional can describe and discuss two or more of the major theories of family development and
psychopathology. *Objective 5(a).* On the basis of his understanding
of family behavior and process, the Mental Health Professional can
apply his knowledge to elicit change in family communication patterns.

Assessment: case presentations; supervisor assessment; tutor
assessment; patient management.

Teaching settings and clinical areas: 2, 7, 9, 10; a–h.

Objective 6. The mental health professional can describe and discuss
the following various theories of group processes and development
(small and large groups; organizations and systems): ethological,
psychoanalytic, NTL, Tavistock, psychodrama, Gestalt, Transactional.

Assessment: supervisor assessment (group); tutor assessment;
patient and group management.

Teaching settings and clinical areas: 2, 5, 8, 9; a–h.

Objective 6(a). The mental health professional demonstrates his
ability to utilize his knowledge of group process to make the necessary interventions to ensure the development of a group.

Assessment: group psychotherapy supervision; tutor assessment; group management.

Teaching settings and clinical areas: 2, 5, 8, 9; a–h.

Psychological and Social Factors

Objective 1. The mental health professional is able to recognize the
specific tasks faced during infancy, childhood, adolescence, early
adulthood, middle age, and old age that are generally assumed to
be a function of these discrete phases of the individual life cycle.

Assessment: case conference presentation; supervisor assessment; tutor assessment.

Teaching settings and clinical areas: 9, 10, 2; a–h.

Objective 2. The mental health professional lists and describes psychiatric or behavioral disorders, both common and rare, associated with each developmental stage.

Assessment: case conference presentation; intake team assessment; patient management.

Teaching settings and clinical areas: 9, 10, 2; a–h.

Objective 3. The mental health professional demonstrates his understanding of the development (from birth to death) of a person over time by relating current problem behaviors to the person's personal and social history.

Assessment: case conference presentation; intake team assessment; supervisor assessment.

Teaching settings and clinical areas: 2, 3, 7, 9; a–h.

Psychiatry and the Law

Objective 1. The mental health professional describes the laws that affect mental patients, such as laws concerned with involuntary hospitalization, responsibility, and drugs.

Assessment: intake team assessment; case presentation.

Teaching settings and clinical areas: 2, 5; a–d, f–h.

Objective 2. The mental health professional discusses the implications of laws for the management of a given psychiatric patient who has been interviewed and examined.

Assessment: intake team assessment; case presentation; patient management.

Teaching settings and clinical areas: 1, 2, 5; a–d, f–h.

Objective 3. The mental health professional can list and utilize the resources of those community agencies which are involved with the legal aspects of community mental health services (juvenile court, legal aid, and so on).

Assessment: intake team assessment; case presentation; patient management.

Teaching settings and clinical areas: 2, 5; a–d, f–h.

Objective 4. The mental health professional uses his knowledge of the laws that affect mental patients to provide satisfactory treatment for his patients.

Assessment: intake team assessment, including emergency room referral; patient management.

Teaching settings and clinical areas: 2, 5, 7; a–d, f–h.

Personal and Professional Growth

Objective 1. The mental health professional demonstrates a willingness to engage in an interworking relationship with other health professionals, as rated by people who work with him daily.

Assessment: supervisor assessment; tutor assessment; periodic review.

Teaching settings and clinical areas: all seminars, especially group development seminars; all clinical experiences.

Objective 2. The mental health professional demonstrates a willingness to work in: (A) a task-oriented group of peers; (B) an interpersonally oriented group of peers; and (C) a task-oriented staff group.

Assessment: supervisor assessment; tutor assessment; periodic review.

Teaching settings and clinical areas: all seminars, especially group development seminars; all clinical experiences.

Objective 3. The mental health professional recognizes and can describe conflicted areas wtihin himself which are elicited by his clinical experiences.

Assessment: supervisor assessment; tutor assessment; periodic review.

Teaching settings and clinical areas: 6, 8, 11; a–h; weekly meeting of trainees with chief resident.

Objective 4. The mental health professional recognizes and can discuss the implications of those feelings produced by his training experience and attempts to understand and use the awareness to develop his personal and professional identity.

Assessment: supervisor assessment; tutor assessment; periodic review.

Teaching settings and clinical areas: 6, 8, 11; trainee meeting; a–h.

Objective 5. The mental health professional demonstrates his awareness of his role in a group situation or a system. *Objective 5(a).* The mental health professional demonstrates a recognition that feelings produced in himself may be a manifestation of the process within his group of peers.

Assessment: supervisor assessment; tutor assessment; periodic review.

Teaching settings and clinical areas: 6, 8, 11; trainee meeting; a–h.

Psychotherapy

Objective 1. The mental health professional demonstrates the ability to (A) listen to a patient; (B) help patients with problems in the psychological and psychiatric area; (C) establish and maintain a working relationship with a patient.

Assessment: orientation evaluation; periodic assessment; supervision; case conference presentation.

Teaching settings and clinical areas: 1, 2, 3, 11; a–d.

Objective 2. The mental health professional describes verbal and nonverbal cues in himself.

Assessment: supervisor evaluation; periodic review; orientation evaluation.

Teaching settings and clinical areas: 1, 11; a–d.

Objective 3. The mental health professional does not permit his own emotional needs to interfere with his responding appropriately to the patient's emotional and physical needs. *Objective 3(a).* The mental health professional is aware of the significance of his own personal background in his reactions to a patient's problem.

Assessment: supervisor evaluation; periodic review; orientation evaluation.

Teaching settings and clinical areas: 1, 11; a–d.

Objective 4. The mental health professional is aware of the significance of his reactions: (A) to failure of his treatment; (B) to the dying patient; (C) to the suicidal or depressed patient; (D) to the demanding or manipulative patient; (E) to the psychotic patient; (F) to the hostile or explosive patient; (G) to the silent, withdrawn patient; (H) to staff needs and expectations of him,

Assessment: supervisor assessment; periodic review; tutor assessment.

Teaching settings and clinical areas: 8, 11; a–d.

Objective 5. The mental health professional, in discussing with his supervisor interviews with any patient, demonstrates that he is aware of the relative merits of his considering and employing alternative ways of responding to the patient.

Assessment: supervisor assessment; case conference presentation; periodic review.

Teaching settings and clinical areas: 1, 3; a–d.

Objective 6. The mental health professional demonstrates that he is able to utilize a conceptual model of psychotherapy in working with his patient. *Objective 6(a).* The mental health professional demonstrates his awareness of the varieties of psychotherapy which are available to him.

Assessment: psychotherapy supervision; case conference presentation.

Teaching settings: 3, 7, 9, 11.

Objective 7. The mental health professional demonstrates that he can effectively use information and feelings communicated to him by the patient to move the patient to a defined therapeutic goal. *Objective 7(a).* The mental health professional is aware of the interaction between him and the patient and can use the interaction to move the patient to defined therapeutic goals.

Assessment: psychotherapy supervision; case conference presentation.

Teaching settings: 3, 7, 9, 11.

Objective 8. The mental health professional demonstrates his awareness of the differences for himself in being a psychotherapist versus being a friend to the patient.

Assessment: psychotherapy supervision; case conference presentation.

Teaching settings: 3, 7, 9, 11.

Social and Community Psychiatry

Objective 1. The mental health professional defines the sociological, cultural, and ethnic factors which are relevant to the work of the

---

mental health team (such as social class, race, systems theory, normality, and illness).

Assessment: participation in seminars; consultation skills.

Teaching settings and clinical areas: 2, 5, 8, 9; a–h.

Objective 2. The mental health professional can list those agencies in the community which provide service relevant to mental health needs.

Assessment: patient management; intake team assessment.

Teaching settings and clinical areas: 2, 5; a–h.

Objective 3. The mental health professional demonstrates his understanding of the basic principles of crisis theory by applying them in clinical settings.

Assessment: intake team assessment; consultation skills; patient management.

Teaching settings and clinical areas: 2, 5, 7, 9; a–h.

Objective 4. From available or elicited data on patients with psychiatric disease, the mental health professional describes the epidemiology (incidence, prevalence, and so on of the diagnosed disorder).

Assessment: intake team assessment; consultation skills.

Teaching settings and clinical areas: 2, 5, 9; a–h.

Objective 5. The mental health professional describes the psychological and social consequences of being subjected to acute and chronic disease.

Assessment: patient management; consultation skills.

Teaching settings and clinical areas: 2, 5, 9; a–h.

Objective 6. The mental health professional describes (based on his analysis) the feasible options a patient has as a function of his age, sex, socioeconomic and cultural status, intelligence, psychopathology, family, and medical condition.

Assessment: patient management; intake team; consultation skills.

Teaching settings and clinical areas: 1, 2, 5, 7, 9; a–h.

Objective 7. Based on an analysis of the patient's life situation, the mental health professional should be able to prescribe at least one treatment regimen for the patient that takes into consideration these factors (that is, his life situation).

Assessment: patient management; intake team; consultation skills.

Teaching settings and clinical areas: 1, 2, 5, 7, 9; a–h.

Objective 8. The mental health professional is able to appropriately state his findings and suggestions to the patient and his family. His response indicates that he has listened to and heard his patient's concern and that he is aware of conflict areas.

Assessment: patient management; intake team; consultation skills.

Teaching settings and clinical areas: 1, 2, 5, 7, 9; a–h.

Objective 9. The mental health professional describes behavioral data which: (A) suggest that an individual is impeded from working effectively (dementia, delirium, thought disorders, anxiety, and depression), and (B) suggest "abnormal illness behavior." He indicates that he understands why referral to or consultation with a psychiatrist was made.

Assessment: patient management; intake team; consultation skills.

Teaching settings: 1, 2, 5, 7, 9.

Objective 10. The mental health professional describes the implications of the differences between his own social and economic background and that of his patients.

Assessment: patient management; intake team assessment; consultation skills.

Teaching settings and clinical areas: 1, 2, 5, 7, 9; a–h.

Objective 11. The mental health professional uses his understanding of group and systems theory and applies this to agency consultation.

Assessment: consultation skills.

Teaching settings and clinical areas: 2, 5, 9; e–h.

Part Five

Funding

AAAAAAAAAAAAAAKKKKKKKKKKKKK

It would be very reasonable to ask why those who train mental health professionals should be concerned with funding treatment programs. Those concerns are more likely to be voiced by practitioners, administrators, and politicians. Yet in reality, it is impossible to divorce training and clinical programs. The education of the health professional is more than reading books or attending seminars. His training is carried on in a clinical setting where actual supervised practice takes place. In addition to providing the necessary patient treatment experience, this setting should be appropriate to the future practice of the psychiatrist or other mental health professional.

The rapid rate of change in health delivery systems suggests that a number of models may evolve during the professional life of today's trainees. The past decade has seen the development of community mental health centers, which will surely expand in numbers and employ many from the manpower pool now in training. The next decade will see the beginning of some kind of national health program. No one doubts that some type of federal legislation will be enacted in the next year or two. Depending upon a number of political considerations, the program may cover catastrophic illness only; it may promote health care delivery by organized groups with prepaid enrollees; it may be a government-administered national

113

health insurance plan. Training programs must prepare mental health professionals to work effectively in these new situations as well as in current settings. This educational responsibility is a major reason for concern with funding clinical programs.

Another reason has to do with the cost of training. Since World War II generous government support of research has had a strong influence on health sciences education. Research support has been a major source of funding and manpower in educational institutions. Training has piggybacked on research. This relationship has not always been advantageous for the educator since research productivity was more likely to be rewarded than teaching.

In addition to the secondary benefits from research, mental health training programs have also received considerable direct government support. With the initiation of the National Institute of Mental Health, Congress has funded training programs in all the mental health professions. The results are apparent in the large increase in mental health manpower. Though that increase has benefited millions of patients, there continues to be a significant shortage of workers in psychiatry, psychology, social work, and nursing. Nevertheless, the Nixon administration has elected to diminish (and has attempted to withdraw) its support for training programs in the mental health professions. Without reciting the arguments or responding to them, today's educator must be keenly aware of the imminent problem he will face in finding funds to carry on training programs.

The reduction of support for training programs and research is accompanied by a major governmental thrust toward increased emphasis on service delivery. If training is not funded by direct subsidy or indirectly by research support then training must benefit from service delivery programs. This necessity is not always welcome news for educators—particularly for medical school faculty, who fear that excessive demands for service will interfere with the teaching and research responsibilities of a university. Nevertheless, a psychiatry department chairman or a mental health training program administrator will be in a better position to involve his program in an appropriate balance of service delivery, teaching, and research if he is familiar with developments now under way.

9

Funding Mental
Health Services

CLAUDEWELL S. THOMAS

HENRY A. FOLEY

Cost, population, and available services are three major characteristics which define the scope of the mental health delivery problem. The annual cost of existing mental health services is at least 4.2 billion dollars. If one looks at the additional costs of patients' lost productivity, another 16 billion dollars should be added. These figures exclude indirect costs of mental illness such as those incurred by criminal behavior associated with drug use and by automobile accidents associated with alcoholism. In terms of population, the lowest estimate is that 10 percent of all people are seriously affected by mental illness at some point in their lives. Children, the aged, and the poor are especially likely to suffer these illnesses. To treat such problems there are many different kinds of service facilities, manpower, and financial support sources, but none of these is currently available either in quantity or quality adequate to treat the mentally ill. Furthermore, those higher quality services which are in operation are maldistributed and therefore not available at all in some population areas. The services are also financially inaccessible to many. Finally, the services are not well enough coordinated with each other and with other health and social service systems to assure appropriate use of mental health resources.

In response to that set of problems, the federal government can and should take action to build a mental health care system which will assure equal access to services, balance the supply of services with the demand for them, organize resources within the system to maximize efficiency, and build on the strengths of those mental health resources already available. There is wide consensus on the need for a delivery system characterized as community-based, comprehensive in scope, and coordinated with other service systems. Such a system should emphasize preventive, early, and ambulatory care and it should be accountable to the public for its services. Serious discussion and debate have commenced on how to finance this system in whole or in phases under national health insurance.

What is most significant in the currently proposed legislative measures is the extent to which individuals with emotional or mental disorders may receive benefits equivalent to other general health benefits. It is uncertain whether equal benefits for mental and physical conditions will be enough to assure the adequacy of mental health services required in a total national health care system. Yet equal benefit status for those with mental disorders is a positive development in the evolution of insurance for mental and emotional disorders. A fundamental criterion for accepting any health insurance proposal must be that mental health care is included as an integral part of the benefit system. The desired financial structure of health care would provide comprehensive coverage of mental health services linked to other human service systems with emphasis on early detection and health maintenance in the community, accessible to all the population, and responsive and accountable to the consumer. Such a system presently does not exist—in part because a public or public-private financing base has yet to be designed which provides equitable financial access to services for all citizens.

The development of the financial conditions to allow real consumer choice will change the delivery of health care services.

The language of all the insurance bills recently proposed in Congress speaks to the need for change, but not all point to a system which provides real choice for all Americans. Although it can be inferred that most of the proposals do indeed include at least some mental health benefits, some bills are in fact discriminatory and regressive in relation to income groups and diagnostic classifications, especially psychiatric diagnosis. The basic issue addressed in this chapter is the need for a financing strategy which supports the benefits of comprehensive mental health services for all citizens in organized service systems.

There are a number of important issues relevant to the evaluation and financing mechanisms of the health system. The first concerns health care resources and their organization. It is obvious that the normal economic controls of the competitive marketplace are not operating in medical care. Rise in prices cannot hold back demand; and the future appears to hold the prospect of increased demands. In the economics of medicine, there is an absence of a market regulator and discipline. And yet certain facts are very clear. The character of financing influences delivery systems and vice versa. The lack of comprehensive coverage causes imbalance and expensive patterns of utilization. In a nation where the population is heterogenous along a multitude of dimensions, where the existing delivery units and facilities are a rich mixture of private, public, nonprofit, proprietary, high quality, and low quality—pushcart vendors along with supermarkets—the effects of a national system of financing and organization improvement are not tractable by "partial equilibrium analysis." We cannot, that is, disaggregate the multitude of possible effects by focusing on just one or two and assuming all other elements equal. We are dealing with a system of many interacting variables, none of whose values can be determined in the absence of the value of the others.

Any discussion of evaluating the total cost of a health system must consider two components: the resources available which affect both direct and indirect costs and the effect on delivery of care of how those resources are organized. The population's capacity to use those resources will inherently depend on the cost to the individual. The total cost of any national health insurance system will be determined by the interaction of the existing availability and organization of resources (resource constraints) and their impact on utilization (satisfied effective demand). Utilization, however, is understood in terms of population and benefit coverage (or exclusion or both) as well as provider attitudes, incentives, quality criteria, levels of pent-up demands, participants' attitudes toward health, the sick role, and the system. Such demographic considerations as the distribution of the population's age, sex, income, and urban-rural residence are also important in the use of medical care.

Historically, mental health care has been chiefly provided through public monies. Because of the development of new treatment modalities and new resources, the cost of psychiatric care is no longer prohibitive. Indeed, it appears that such care may reduce the overall utilization of general medical resources. As a result, in the last two decades such care increasingly has been included in health insurance plans. At present, psychiatric care is financed predominantly through the following modes of payment: public funds, personal income and savings, and partial subsidy through insurance or prepayment plans. According to Reed (1972), about 134 million people or 67 percent of the population had some coverage for physicians' in-hospital visits for general illness; for mental conditions, about 108 million people or 54 percent of the population had some coverage for such visits. About 86.3 million persons or 43 percent of the population had some coverage for physicians' office visits for general illness; whereas about 73 million or 63.5 percent of the population had some coverage for office visits related to mental conditions. Those persons with some coverage of care for mental illness comprise about 80 percent of the total of all who have health insurance for any illness—be it for hospital care, physicians' in-hospital visits, or physicians' office visits. While recognizing that the mental illness coverage is often meager, we think these figures settle once and for all the question of whether insurance coverage of mental illness is feasible. How could it *not* be feasible when it is so widespread?

We will first describe a desirable national insurance package which includes definite mental health benefits and then discuss the implications of national health insurance for medical education, undergraduate, graduate, and postgraduate. The optimal level of medical care in relation to mental illness should cover prevention, active treatment (both inpatient and outpatient), rehabilitation, and long-term care and collateral services to families of the mentally ill. There should be no limitations as to age, sex, or condition. Any limits on mental health services should be determined by regulations based on clinical experience—the scientific base—and subject to approval of citizens' boards—the consumer input.

There are nine clusters of impact tendencies supported by current federal policy in the mental health fields which should be strengthened and not weakened by a national insurance program.

Toward organized systems of care (away from fragmented services). Fragmented care in the mental health field means that patients experience difficulty in transferring from one modality of care or facility to another when such changes are indicated. For example, intensive inpatient care may take place without adequate follow-up and result in rehospitalization. Intensive outpatient care may be followed by totally discontinuous varieties of state hospital care. Organized systems of care should provide continuity. The parts of the system should be clearly articulated with boundaries and functions well defined, with the goal of smooth patient flow.

A second function of an organized care system is to examine itself and commit services in needed areas. Metaphorically, one might consider a battle in which each soldier does what in good conscience seems best to him in contrast to an organized army system whose commanders commit their troops to the areas where they are most needed and shift their supplies accordingly. An organized system of care can develop multidisciplinary teams, comprehensive services, early detection programs, outpatient services, close linkages with other human service systems, and accountability to the consumer and can expand the availability and accessibility of all services in a meaningful pattern. Thus, an organized system of care often seems a prerequisite to the remaining eight desirable tendencies.

In examining national health insurance plans one should look for the possibility of "front-end" (preventive services) funding or other incentives needed to create such comprehensive care systems. Creating successful inter- and intra-organizational care systems takes time, energy, and money in "boundary maintenance" and "observing ego" (consumer evaluation) functions. Specifically, these activities require conference and thinking time. When insurance recompenses solo practitioners on an equal basis with a care system, the total salaries in the care system tend to be less. Because the flow gradient is toward solo practice among graduating psychiatric residents and among people given unrestricted purchasing power for psychiatric services, insurance plans which do not in some way discriminate against fee-for-service payments may well prove disruptive to an organized care system. Plans should be examined for their potential in providing incentives to such an approach.

Toward a multidisciplinary approach (away from exclusive reliance on physicians). Some of the costs involved in developing organized care systems may be ameliorated by emphasizing use of many disciplines. Psychiatric nurses, social workers, psychologists, mental health counselors, mental health technicians, rehabilitation counselors, occupational therapists, recreational therapists cost less than physicians per unit of time; provide a great range of skills beyond the limits of any single physician; and, most important, provide a potentially mobile pool of mental health manpower. Even if the multidisciplinary approach did not provide additional skills at lower costs, it would still be necessary because of the shortage of physicians trained in psychiatry.

The multidisciplinary team should be emphasized. The issues of standard-setting and regulation of solo practice have proved virtually unsolvable even among trained physicians. To extend these problems to health professionals with less stringent traditions of self-regulation would seem very undesirable. Thus, each health insurance proposal should be examined to see whether it fosters payments to physicians only, payments to organized teams, or fee-for-service payments to allied health professionals. It would be best if payments were made to physicians or organized group facilities which could utilize the services of other disciplines. Standards for organized facilities should be left to regulations established by the Secretary of Health, Education, and Welfare.

Toward comprehensive services for mental health (away from limited services for mental illness). The concept of comprehensive services is intended to foster a variety of approaches responsive to the needs of individuals, families, and communities. Specifically, plans should be analyzed to see whether they depend on rigid use of diagnostic categories of "mental disease" and whether they make any provision for consultative and educational services. Most health insurance has been willing to cover general medical care for a variety of presenting symptoms related to "the stress of living." Paradoxically, mental health services (the services appropriate to such problems) are often excluded. Contrary to fears within the insurance industry, experience with the United Automobile Workers' plan thoroughly demonstrates that providing services for a variety of family dysfunctions (such as marital problems, adjustment reactions in adolescence, school problems) does not result in overutilization. The different national insurance proposals vary in their provisions from a broad range of comprehensive health services to a more narrow group of "severe illness" services.

Toward early detection, health maintenance (away from delayed treatment of illness). As we have already indicated, traditional insurance programs tend to avoid commitment to comprehensive services. Specifically, the comprehensive services most likely to be excluded are those with maximal social desirability (early detection and prevention). At a minimum, early detection of illness is desirable to diminish patient suffering and family disruption. In many fields of medicine, early case detection tends to diminish severity and long-term disability. This tendency is *probably* true in psychiatry and mental health. As practical programs in prevention become available in the coming decades, the national health insurance system should foster their implementation.

For programs of health maintenance and prevention of illness, front end funding is a necessity. Pure fee-for-service arrangements tend to discourage such programs. The critical variables in early detection coverage are the elimination of deductible amounts, minimal co-insurance, and front-end funding for mental health services. High deductibles are designed to ensure that insurance benefits are only used for catastrophic illness. This result may be a "self-fulfilling prophecy" in that treatment is delayed (because of financial barriers) until illness has reached catastrophic proportions. The financial disincentive to early treatment is likely to discourage treatment in lower income groups even where it is necessary and to have no effect in high-income groups. There is no evidence that deductibles screen out inappropriate utilizers, only those without money.

Toward encouraging outpatient services (away from hospitalization incentives). The current insurance practice of deemphasizing outpatient mental health services through limitations, exclusions, or high co-insurance payments is extremely undesirable. Such an approach encourages a physician to use the most expensive form of treatment available, because it will cost his patient the least. Illnesses may go untreated until hospitalization is necessary. In other cases inappropriate use of hospital beds may be fostered. Available evidence indicates that adding outpatient benefits markedly reduces the cost per patient treated. Where regular outpatient care is not possible, other nonhospital care, such as day care, halfway houses, residential schools, foster home placements, and so on, should be encouraged. Whether a variety of treatment modalities *not* employing traditional hospital beds can be funded will determine the extent of payments for nonhospital care.

Toward encouraging close linkages with other human services (away from exclusive ties to health systems). There are a whole series of boundaries which the mental health disciplines share with other human services. The mental health care system of the future may be increasingly dependent upon ties to the general educational system, the social welfare system, the recreational system, industrial units (employers and unions), the law enforcement system, and others. Mental health services have not fared well when left under the exclusive control of general physicians. States in which mental health services are buried in health departments have often lagged behind in developing mental health services, compared to states with discrete mental health authorities. General health care plans which do not specify any separate mental health organizational components have tended to ignore mental health issues and to confine their activities to limited psychiatric consultation and evaluation. Thus, if comprehensive health units are specified and no provision is made for community mental health units, linkages with other units may suffer. Currently proposed national insurance plans vary in their provision of relationships between the general health system and other human services. The organizational framework of a program tends to create these relationships.

Toward public responsiveness and accountability (away from prime concern for health providers and their financiers). Responsiveness, accountaibility, and sensitivity to consumer needs provide crucial feedback information for program modification. Health professionals and financiers have tended to dominate the boards of voluntary health insurance organizations. The community mental health center system has been set up to attempt to ensure feedback from consumers of mental health care.

Toward expanding the availability and accessibility of all services. Accessibility of mental health services is contingent upon two elements: consumer factors, and facility factors. The main consumer factors are information about the availability of the service, the psychological-educational readiness to employ such a service, the financial means to use the service, and the geographic proximity of the service. Facility factors include availability of personnel to man the service, existence of waiting lists, and physical facilities. Some resource and geographic limitations can be overcome by paying transportation costs. Insurance plans which rely on fragmented fee-for-service care systems will tend to foster waiting lists and limited accessibility to all forms of service.

Toward coverage for the total population (away from limited coverage). The plans that cover broad population groups without regard to economic status or other special characteristics will tend to promote equitable access to mental health care. On the other hand, insurance "packages" designed separately for low-income groups, the poor, the "uninsurables," the aged, and so on will help preserve fragmented double standards of care and limited access to services. If employment is the main entitlement, it is possible that some groups may be excluded from coverage.

The NIMH Task Force on National Health Insurance developed a number of criteria for optional mental health insurance plans. The primary emphasis is on the prevention and early detection of incipient illness and removal of financial and psychological barriers to utilization of appropriate resources. As such, the optional plan provides a "system(s) designed adequately to meet the mental health needs of the American people."

Evaluation (including diagnostic and referral services) should be protected by unlimited coverage. The emphasis should be on the development of mental health evaluation services in organized health care settings and the importance of mental health evaluation as a component of general health care. Benefits should include psychiatric evaluation, psychological testing, and other procedures to determine medical disability.

Inpatient benefits should be provided as needed but not emphasized. They should not be differentiated from general health benefits. In order to qualify, a patient should be in active treatment under an individualized treatment plan. Benefits for inpatients should not be more generous than outpatient benefits. Service could be provided in qualified general hospitals, community mental health centers, or psychiatric hospitals. If care is anticipated beyond ninety days, prior authorization should be obtained.

Outpatient benefits should include unlimited coverage for services of a multidisciplinary team in organized mental health settings (providers). Private practitioners would be required to have affiliation agreements with organized mental health settings in order to have available appropriate evaluation, partial hospitalization, and rehabilitation sources. Individual therapy, group therapy, and family therapy should be included. Length of treatment should be determined by peer review mechanisms.

Partial hospitalization programs should provide alternatives to inpatient care. They can be offered by qualified mental health providers in a nonhospital setting. Unlimited coverage should be given, but prior authorization should be obtained for care to continue beyond eighteen days. Programs should have a hospital linkage in order to provide twenty-four–hour care.

Rehabilitation services should include full coverage as prescribed by approved mental health providers according to specific requirements of individual treatment plans. Counseling and case consultation should be included for the patient and the family and for employee and other significant rehabilitation referral agencies.

Extended care should provide sixty to ninety days' coverage per "spell of illness" in a qualified mental health transitional facility such as a halfway house. It might also be provided in a unit capable of offering adequate psychosocial care. Benefits should provide two days of care in a social facility in exchange for one day of hospitalization. They should be offered on the basis of an individualized treatment plan for each patient.

Home health services should provide unlimited visits of

mental health teams based on a treatment plan. There should be emphasis on collaborative services offered by mental health providers and general health providers. Homemakers' services should be included.

Prescription drugs should be completely covered for both inpatients and outpatients. The drugs should be available through a generic formulary according to federal standards.

Community-based, multidiscipline peer review (including consumer participation) teams should provide assessment in prepaid, organized settings for all mental health services. A history of prior hospitalization should be required before a patient gets reimbursement for "long-term" psychotherapy. Specialized criteria should be developed for mental health services.

Services of all mental health personnel, including psychiatric social workers, clinical psychologists, psychiatric nurses, occupational therapists, physical therapists, and rehabilitation therapists, should be available through mental health providers or through other approved, organized settings.

Whatever the eventual resolution of national health insurance issues, educational functions will be affected significantly by current federal programs, including Medicare, Medicaid, and CHAMPUS (an insurance plan for military dependents). Other programs include health center programs and medical research and training grants. A continuous assessment and evaluation of these programs must occur and must be shared with all physicians. Some initial directions are now indicated from the debate around national health insurance. There will clearly be a greater focus on community medicine. Consequently, preventive and community medicine should get increased attention in medical education. These skills should include training in and understanding of the consultative process as well as experience in relationships with allied professions.

Use of rehabilitative workers and members of related disciplines will certainly be emphasized. Physicians now need to be trained in such a way that they do not disparage the skills of vocational rehabilitation workers, so that they rely on these skilled staff to develop rehabilitation programs, and so that they become cautious about removing the patient from his world of work in order to cure him. To develop this perspective, the curriculum of the medical school must incorporate training in the field of vocational rehabilitation to develop students' understanding of and respect for the vocational model. Enough studies in this country and elsewhere have demonstrated the therapeutic value of work.

As a consequence of changes in Medicare and Medicaid there will certainly be a greater interface between mental health workers and other medical personnel. This change will surely require greater emphasis on supervised interprofessional learning in all fields. The demands of new programs will make it essential to increase all types of mental health manpower. In such times, any national health insurance program should promote the use of existing psychiatric facilities for educational purposes.

Impact of National
Health Insurance

WALTER E. BARTON

※※※※※※※※※※※※※※※ﾑﾑﾑﾑﾑﾑﾑﾑﾑﾑﾑﾑ

*I*s it economically feasible for
an insurance program to cover an acute episode of mental illness
on the same basis as physical illness? What is the average length of
stay in hospital for a psychiatric disorder? What is the rate of use
of in-bed facilities for psychiatric disorders? Can most patients with
a mental illness be treated as outpatients? If so, how many outpatient sessions are required on the average? What is the cost of
inpatient and outpatient services for mental illness as compared to
the cost for service for other illnesses?

The American Psychiatric Association set out, some years
ago, to get the answers to these questions. Ten years ago, the APA
was joined by the National Association for Mental Health and
Group Health Insurance, Inc., of New York in a study of psychiatric insurance, reported in a book by Helen Avnet (1962). The
principal findings included the demonstration that psychiatrists were
available to service patients who needed help; that different sub-
groups in the population varied widely in their use of psychiatric

benefits; that utilization rates decreased after initial backlog of demand was satisfied. There was a trend toward earlier treatment as the project continued. The patients who sought help needed it. Insurance coverage for acute mental illness proved feasible. The APA-NAMH Joint Information Service, in 1962 and again in 1967, surveyed the extent of insurance coverage for mental disorders and published *Health Insurance for Mental Illness* (Scheidemandel, Kanno, and Glasscote, 1967).

In 1963, the president-elect of the American Psychiatric Association, Daniel Blain, had luncheon with Melvin A. Glasser, director of the Social Security Department of the United Automobile, Aerospace, and Agricultural Implement Workers of America (UAW). Glasser indicated, during the conversation, that UAW intended to bargain for fringe benefits that included improved prepaid insurance. Blain suggested that the benefit package include coverage for psychiatric disorders. This conversation led to a series of exchanges which were ultimately negotiated in 1964 labor-management contracts with the automobile industry. APA representatives actually consulted with both labor and management in the negotiating process.

In 1965, the National Association of Private Psychiatric Hospitals and the National Association of State Mental Health Program Directors joined with the APA in a workshop on "Psychiatric Issues in Insurance." The goal of the workshop was to plan a national congress on psychiatric insurance. At that time I suggested that before a national congress was held many policy issues needed resolution. As a consequence of this suggestion, a series of propositional statements were prepared by the APA staff and several two-day workshops were held in 1965, with intervening homework. The product of these workshops became the first edition of APA *Guidelines for Psychiatric Services Covered under Health Insurance Plans* that was to have such a profound influence on the field. Many organizations worked with the APA to develop these guidelines. Among them were the National Institute of Mental Health, the American Medical Association, the National Association of Private Psychiatric Hospitals, the National Association of State Mental Health Program Directors, and the Michigan Health and Social Security Research Institute. A series of informal conferences followed, with representatives of labor, management, and insurance carriers, in order that the provisions of the guidelines might be incorporated in policy and action.

Also in 1965, the AMA held its 11th Annual Conference of State Mental Health Representatives, which devoted half a day to the subject of health insurance. This conference provided an opportunity to involve all of medicine in the progress toward including coverage for psychiatric disorders in any insurance benefit plan. The APA also at this time called together medical specialty and mental health professional organizations to support accreditation as a standard for inclusion in Medicare legislation, and the APA worked actively to modify the Medicare amendments to provide basic psychiatric benefits. These goals were accomplished.

Study of UAW Plan and Other Psychiatric Insurance

The inclusion of a psychiatric benefit in the UAW program made it possible to examine the use of services among blue-collar workers. The APA jointly secured a grant with the Michigan Health and Social Security Research Institute for a study in three phases. Phase One began on June 1, 1965, and continued for two years. The project operated with two teams. In the Washington office, I was the project director, assisted by Robert Pfeiller. In the Detroit office, Glasser was the co-director, aided by Karl Girshman and Thomas McPartland. During this phase, district branches of the APA were involved in establishing a service network that could support the benefits of the program. Visits were made to some seventy-seven cities where most UAW workers were concentrated. In Michigan, preutilization studies were made and a system of reporting was set up. Many substudies were suggested that included such topics as: general hospital management compared with management in other psychiatric facilities; the effect of health education on utilization rates; the effectiveness of treatment as determined by the number of work days lost by reason of mental illness; the cost of psychiatric benefits and of other medical benefits; the effectiveness of the plan in meeting needs under a dollar limit; the patterns of use and costs of services in different health delivery systems; and the extent of service benefits for psychiatric disorders when given by other than psychiatrists. At the end of Phase One, the project had achieved many of its original objectives. The profession responded with interest and organized the required services to deliver the agreed benefits.

During this period insurance coverage for psychiatric illness had been growing. Many related study projects had developed within the field, such as psychiatric care among union workers at Johns Hopkins; problems in insuring for psychiatric services at the University of California at Berkeley; benefit programs for workers in mental health at Roosevelt University; mental health rehabilitation for a union population in New York City; utilization of medical services by Group Health Insurance in Washington, D.C.

Phase Two was exclusively the responsibility of the UAW, and the APA discontinued its participation in the project. The report of the findings of this study, it is anticipated, will be published in book form by the UAW. Glasser (1972) writes:

Under the UAW program, the covered person paid nothing for the first five visits to a private psychiatrist; 15% of the physician's fee for the sixth through tenth visit; 30% for the eleventh through the fifteenth visit; and 45% thereafter, until a maximum of $400 in claims had been utilized. No co-payment is required if the patient receives service from an organized health services program such as a prepaid group practice plan or an approved mental health center. The program, at its conclusion, covered nearly 3 million workers, including members of their families.

The experience of the UAW in Michigan was studied intensively by the project staff of the Michigan Health and Social Security Research Institute. During 1967, from among approximately 1 million eligible persons in Michigan, 8,500 made use of the psychiatric benefit. In 1968, this rose to 11,500, and to over 14,000 in 1969. The numbers are not cumulative but refer to the number of persons using the benefit within a calendar year. This mode of reporting was necessary because the $400 maximum is renewed for each member of the eligible population on the first day of the year.

In terms of rates, these figures represent 7.7 per 1,000 eligibles in 1967; 9.8 in 1968; and 11.3 in 1969. This indicates a gradual

*increase in each successive year's study, with the rate surpassing the
1% level in the final year of study. For the most part, these users
of services received their treatment in the private sector. In 1967,
about 60% of those who needed treatment were in a private practice
setting. In 1968, this rose to about 70% and in 1969 surpassed
75%. This was in spite of the co-payment factor required and applicable in private practice. It was also noted that the organized group
facilities serviced a relatively constant number of UAW eligibles
each year. The prevailing mode of treatment was the full session,
1 hour of individual psychotherapy. About three-fourths of the users
of service in each year were served this form of treatment.*

*In terms of averages each year, approximately 7 services
were received by the users of benefits. The $400 maximum benefit is
also a matter of interest. In 1967 and in 1968, only about 4% of
those who used this benefit reached that limit. Thus, about 96%
appeared to have been adequately served within the limit. In 1969,
almost 9% used the full limit of the benefit.*

*The rate of hospitalization remained constant—4.7 per
1,000—in 1965, a year prior to the inauguration of the outpatient
benefit, and for 1967 and 1968, after the new benefits were available, indicating that hospitalization for mental conditions did not
decrease when the outpatient benefit was made available."*

Phase Three of the study project, reported in Reed, Myers,
and Scheidmandel (1972), examined data about psychiatric benefits in many different plans. The report includes the Canadian experience in some detail; the nearly five million persons covered under
federal employees' benefit insurance programs; the Blue Cross-Blue
Shield experience; commercial carriers; Kaiser-Permanente; and
many others. Consultants in the insurance field, including a few
knowledgeable psychiatrists, examined the data and added their
interpretations. Field visits were made by experts, when necessary,
and computer runs were made specially for the project. The report
is the most extensive compilation of psychiatric insurance data thus
far available. In the following pages I extract a few summarizing
statements to indicate the nature of the data.

How to pay for medical care has always been a problem
except for the wealthy. Because of the problem of payment for cata-

strophic illness, most individuals requiring long-term care found this service in public mental hospitals. In 1910, 96 percent of all hospitalized mental patients were in long-term hospitals. By 1920, child guidance clinics had developed, and in the 1930s general hospital sections of psychiatry were being revived with increasing emphasis on the use of electric shock therapy and insulin treatment. In the 1950s, psychotropic drugs and a revolution in patient management made it possible to release many patients from mental hospitals, to shorten the stay in hospital, and to extend extramural care. In the 1960s, the community mental health program developed with the help of federal funding for staffing and construction. So radical were the changes that for the first time more patients were being admitted to general hospital psychiatric sections than to all mental hospitals combined. Therefore, the study of psychiatric benefits under insurance plans was made against the backdrop of dramatic changes in the care system.

In 1940, only 12 million persons in the United States had protection against the cost of hospital care through private insurance. By 1969, 157 million, approximately three-fourths of the population, had such protection; while in that same year, 86.3 million, or 43 percent of the covered population, had some coverage for physicians' services in the office and at home. Also, one out of every three beds in the United States was a psychiatric bed. Of these, 413,000 were in state and county mental hospitals (310 institutions); 38,000 were in Veterans Administration neuropsychiatric hospitals (34); 14,000 in private mental hospitals (152); and 22,394 in general hospitals (663). In 1970, there were 275 community mental health centers in operation and 408 had been funded. In 1969, the operating community mental health center programs handled 372,000 admissions and serviced 76,000 inpatients.

In 1955, there were two and a half times as many patients in mental hospitals as in treatment in outpatient departments. By 1968, there were 500,000 more patients receiving treatment in outpatient departments than in mental hospitals. Similarly, this change is marked by a dramatic decline in the inpatient census. In 1955, there were 559,000 patients in mental hospitals and in 1970 the number had dropped to 339,000. In 1971 the drop was 8.5 percent from the previous year. In 1956, total admissions to mental hospitals for psychiatric illness were 185,500; by 1970 total admissions had increased to 393,200. In other words, the drop in census in mental hospitals occurred along with a dramatic increase in admissions of about 112 percent. Discharges had increased during this same span of approximately fifteen years by 175 percent. For example, in 1970, 539,000 patients were discharged from general hospital psychiatric units with a psychiatric diagnosis. In 1970, 2,088 outpatient departments were counted and in the year previous they handled 881,000 patient admissions. Fifty-four percent of inpatient care was handled in less than thirty days in 1969, and in that year, 41 percent of inpatient care cases were handled in under fourteen days.

The cost in 1968 to the citizens of the United States for mental illness and its treatment plus the loss of earnings, according to an NIMH study, was $21 billion. $17 billion was due to loss of productive capacity through inability to work and $4 billion was the cost of treatment. An examination of who paid this cost revealed that 43 percent was borne by state and local governments; 25 percent by the federal government; 18 percent by families; and 12 percent by private sources. Private insurance paid 54 percent of the costs in general hospitals and 52 percent of the costs in private mental hospitals. The average, daily maintenance expenditure per resident patient in a public mental hospital in that year was $14.89. A day of care in a VA hospital in 1970 cost $30 and in a general hospital an average of $81.

All seventy-four Blue Cross plans (July 1971) provided some coverage for mental conditions for some of their subscribers. Out of the 73.5 million subscribers, 82 percent were under group contracts. Benefits for mental illness care in general hospitals, under the most widely held contracts, are less extensive than for other illnesses. For example, in the most commonly held plan, Blue Cross-Blue Shield provided 120 to 125 days of coverage for general illness, but only 30 to 31 days for mental illness. Eighteen plans excluded care in a private mental hospital and forty plans excluded care in public mental hospitals. Under the most widely held contract, thirty-three Blue Cross plans cover alcoholic patients without limitation on days of care, but nineteen plans limit the days and twenty-two exclude care of alcoholic patients altogether. The situation is similar for drug addiction. Self-inflicted injuries are excluded in four plans but

134 Mental Health Education in New Medical Schools

covered in seventy-one. There is an interesting variation in inpatient days, which are high for mental illness when all admissions for all illnesses are high and low for mental illness when admissions for all other illnesses are low.

There has been a reluctance to cover mental illness in such plans, largely due to the number of patients in state mental hospitals and the prolonged stay that has characterized their care in the past. Standards of care were also of concern. In the past few years, private mental hospitals have made a determined drive to improve standards, and presently more than two-thirds are accredited by the Joint Commission on Accreditation of Hospitals.

Group prepayment plans tended to have lower hospital utilization rates. In the group prepayment plans, when the days of care were 365 days per confinement for general illnesses, they were the same for mental illness in general hospitals and in member mental hospitals. About half of all private mental hospitals were member hospitals but there were few public hospitals so classified. The days of care were 69.8 per 1,000 population covered, or 7.1 percent of the total days for all illnesses. The average inhospital stay was 16.3 days for an episode of mental illness as against an average inhospital stay of 7.5 days for all other illnesses.

The Aetna Insurance Company data indicate that 15 percent and 10 percent of all inpatient stay time was for mental illness. Charges per day for mental illness were about two-thirds of those for other illnesses. The lower per diem charges offset the longer stay of the mentally ill.

Payments for physicians' inhospital care of psychiatric patients were 9.7 percent of total claims paid under high option plans and 6.4 percent under low option plans for all conditions. Payments for outpatient services in high option plans were 6.2 percent of all costs for mental disorders; in low option plans, 6.3 percent. The outpatient care benefit required a deductible of one hundred dollars and visits were limited to twenty. The costs in 1970 for physicians' services for outpatient care were two dollars per covered person under either a high or low option plan. In summary, the total annual cost for psychiatric benefits amounted to seven dollars per covered individual, with two dollars for physicians' services in extramural settings, $0.64 for physicians' services in hospital, and the remainder for the cost of services in hospital.

The Kaiser-Permanente plans showed that 91 percent of patients with mental disorders were managed in twenty visits or less. If fifty visits were covered, only 1 percent of the covered population would be eliminated from benefits.

In the Medicare plan, which covers nine million persons sixty-five years of age or over, with no limit on days of care in a general hospital but a 190-day limitation in a lifetime in a psychiatric hospital, psychiatric diagnosis accounted for 1.4 percent of all discharges; days of care for mental disorders were 1.6 percent of all days; the length of stay for all patients was 12.9 days and for psychiatric patients 15.1 days. The cost for psychiatric services was 0.7 percent of all costs inhospital, and the cost per one thousand covered population was $1.69 for psychiatric illness. Increased use of general hospitals rather than mental hospitals by Medicare patients for psychiatric diagnosis was reported.

In the CHAMPUS program, which covers dependents of individuals on active duty with the armed forces, 4.4 percent of admissions to civilian hospitals were for mental disorders, including personality problems. For the retired, the percentage of the total admissions for mental disorders was higher: 10.9 percent.

Since 1958, Canada has had a federal insurance program in which the government pays 50 percent of the cost. Admissions for mental illness were 4.7 per 1,000 population. These patients had a utilization rate of 83.4 days per 1,000 covered population, and the average stay was 17.6 days. The average payment for psychiatric services in 1969 was $10.63, and 54 percent of this sum went to general practitioners for their services to patients.

Several conclusions may be derived from this study. Citizens need health insurance that covers mental illness, for it spreads the risk of heavy expense for medical care. No health service can be considered complete without coverage for psychiatric disorders. Presently, available health insurance benefits for mental illness fall far short of the desirable. Emphasis presently is on inpatient care. The cost of a day of care on the psychiatric service is less than for other illnesses, but more days are required for psychiatric illnesses.

However, the low utilization rate and the offsetting lower bed costs make it feasible to cover inpatient services for psychiatric patients. It appears that coverage of twenty sessions will meet the need of 90 percent of persons who require outpatient services.

The UAW benefit plan, without deductibles, brings patients into treatment early in the course of illness. The service is not excessively used. Full coverage of hospital care and of physicians' in-hospital service is feasible for mental illness on the same basis as for other illnesses. Short-term, outpatient coverage benefit payments are feasible. When the total number of sessions is limited to twenty or less, the cost is but two dollars per year. It is suggested that the benefit plan provide twenty sessions followed by peer review, and if further treatment is imperative, twenty more sessions be funded, as this addition will satisfy the requirements of most of the population.

The population-at-risk that may increase costs is the young, the educated, and those receiving long-term psychotherapy and psychoanalysis. The present restrictions and limitations on psychiatric benefits (that is, no coverage or fewer days for mental illness, and restricted coverage in private and public hospitals when they are approved by the Joint Commission on Accreditation of Hospitals) should be removed.

Impact on Services

It is axiomatic that service follows the dollar. Strange things may occur. For example, if national health insurance were to exclude psychiatrists and cover all other physicians, as one of the national health insurance plans before Congress presently provides, it would not be surprising to find all psychiatrists quickly reidentifying themselves as physicians.

Accreditation is now essential for qualification for benefits in some plans. Some plans favor the general hospital. When coverage extends to private mental hospitals they will serve more of the population.

When extramural care is covered and when freedom of choice is given to the patient, most will choose the care of a psychiatrist in private practice in preference to an organized treatment facility. (More than 75 percent of UAW workers received treatment in a physician's office even though they had to pay a co-insurance benefit and had a limitation on the number of funded treatments— restrictions which did not apply in an organized setting.) If organized services are covered, community mental health programs may be expected to treat more patients. Most HMOs presently funded as experimental programs offer little, if any, psychiatric services.

Impact on Educational Programs

Usually the acute illness receives the most attention from the student in training and from the sponsoring faculty as well. However, students need also to learn the management of chronic diseases, including mental illness. Community mental health programs and their extramural services for drug abuse, alcoholism, and for children offer a stimulating new field for instruction. The general hospital system, with its outpatient department and emergency service, is extensively utilized. Students need to acquire experience in settings likely to be relevant to their mode of practice.

Private practice is a viable health service delivery system and the blue-collar worker prefers it when funded under a group plan. Private care may even be less expensive per hour of service than service in some organized settings.

Today, the economics of health care is a most legitimate curriculum addition. The withdrawal of all federal support for psychiatric training is threatened. The hard-won victory of 1971, approved by Congress, and finally by the Office of Management and Budget, is not the end of the campaign. Policy change is still under consideration and will again suggest withdrawal of federal support for training of mental health professionals. Alternate methods for financing residency training in psychiatry must be studied. It is alleged that we must receive support as do other medical specialists. Perhaps a charge might be made for services performed by residents and add this to bed care costs. Residents might be required to pay a fee for training costs out of the income received for services to patients. Bed costs might be increased, as another alternative, to the point where the hospital's income is sufficient to pay stipends to trainees at the level paid residents in other medical specialties.

Teaching costs might be met through federal support of another approach. A student loan program is possible, although previous studies have rejected it for many reasons. Regional training centers, supported in part by federal funds, have been suggested by other studies and remain a possibility.

There is little doubt that there will be a national health insurance plan, not next year, perhaps, but in the years ahead. Any plan should provide protection for the citizens of this country for mental illness as well as for other illnesses. Detailed studies have demonstrated that it is feasible to cover both inpatient and outpatient care costs for mental illness.

Discussion

The resource papers by Barton and Thomas initiated an active and helpful clarification of issues and highlighted questions which could not yet be answered. The major issues are subsumed under the topical headings in this chapter.

Trends in Mental Health Delivery Systems

Mental health professionals are dealing with the political process, which is not necessarily rational. Problems in service delivery are being obscured by the current funding difficulties. A number of current proposals are offered on the supposition that they will constitute better care for less money. The reality is that quality comprehensive health care is going to cost more money than is currently being spent. The nine impact tendencies described by Thomas may be seen as movements toward change and redefinition of psychiatric matters. Over a period of time these tendencies may result in a redefinition of psychiatry and of the other mental health professions. Those concerned with quality health care are moving toward a system which emphasizes continuity of care and comprehensive service. This system seems to be the only way to have preventative

139

services included. Taking a multidisciplinary team approach means that the funding system must be able to reimburse other mental health professionals in addition to these psychiatrists. Some groups may be funded through the physician, although it is clear that the service delivery system of the future will require a team of mental health professionals. A tendency toward truly comprehensive services requires mental health to be broadly defined and not limited by categorical illnesses which occur in a single individual. Another aspect of comprehensiveness is the fact that services must be community-based and the community must be involved in defining service. Another trend supports prevention and true health maintenance, going beyond early detection of disease. It will require a conscious effort on the part of psychiatry to further develop expertise which can be applied to other parts of human services or human welfare systems. This approach requires that mental health professionals involve themselves in welfare systems, public schools, and the criminal justice system. Ambulatory or outpatient care is increasing for reasons of economy and avoiding social disability. The goals of ambulatory care must emphasize functioning rather than the regression or hospitalism which are the results of custodial or institutional care. We are also moving toward a multiservice system linkage and away from narrow categorical illnesses which define specific health services. The trend toward greater community responsiveness and ultimately community definition of health services is a touchy and difficult area, and there is no reason to believe that communities can accomplish this without education and guidance. Increased accessability of services is tied to the previously mentioned need to develop multiservice or human service systems. The movement toward population coverage means that those mental health services which are developed must be responsible to a specific population and not just to those who come seeking help because of episodic acute illness.

All these trends will require redefinitions of the notion of primary responsibility of each individual for his own health care and of individual determinism of health and illness, success or failure. A sense of social responsibility must be developed in order to interfere with those factors which produce illness and failure. A major shift in training, will be needed to emphasize learning how to prevent disability as well as how to treat illness. Such a shift on the part of psychiatrists will require a reeducation of the community as well as of mental health professionals.

Mental Illness and National Health Insurance

Barton's chapter points to the necessity for including coverage for mental illness under national health insurance. Any national health program which excludes mental health is certainly not truly a health program. That fact is self-evident, but mental health professionals seem to have to battle continuously for such an obvious basic principle. There continues to be public stigma about mental illness. The federal government exhibits a curious schizophrenia, cutting psychiatric benefits in the federal employees' plan while at the same time demonstrating that mental health treatment works. There is a myth that goes all the way back to the 1930s when social security legislation was first written. Mental illness and tuberculosis were excluded because they were treated in public institutions and funded elsewhere. It was assumed that the federal government should not pay for that which is already funded in another fashion. Another common argument is that mental illness coverage is too expensive. This claim has been exploded with hard facts from government research and also with the data which the American Psychiatric Association has accumulated. Nevertheless, there continues to be a real reeducative challenge—a challenge to prove that psychiatric coverage is desirable and economically feasible. Prepaid plans assume that someone else will pay (usually the government), and the federal government assumes that the states will take care of mental illness. We have not yet convinced the nation that most mental illness can be treated in the community in spite of the fact that the state hospital population has diminished drastically and community programs have demonstrated their ability to treat and rehabilitate patients successfully. Most prepaid plans have excluded or markedly limited coverage for mental illness on grounds of insufficient demand and excessive costs, stating that the government is doing it anyway.

The discussants highlighted the fact that existing proposals for national health insurance either eliminate or severely restrict coverage for mental disorder. The Administration proposal specifically excludes services provided by psychiatrists. The other proposals either discriminate against those with mental disorder by sharply limiting benefits or, when they do provide equal coverage, limit the overall program so that effective treatment programs could not be provided under such a plan. Most proposals emphasize inpatient rather than ambulatory care.

Barton reported how the APA wanted to examine all of the experience of insurance plans and prepaid group practice plans. The APA looked at forty different plans and made special computer runs to get data. In addition to the Canadian experience, it studied the federal employee benefit program under which 4.7 million people are covered. Blue Cross and Blue Shield (with seventy-six different plans) made available data from their experience, as did Kaiser-Permanente (the oldest and most representative health maintenance organization—HMO). The APA study, led by Reed, assembled data into tables, and a group of highly experienced consultants such as insurance companies' vice presidents, national insurance council consultants, and other experts in health economics, analyzed the results. That study (the Reed Report) is the most comprehensive single collection of data about psychiatric care and health insurance. It clearly demonstrated the economic feasibility of including coverage for mental illness under national health insurance programs.

It was also pointed out that several states, such as Connecticut, Massachusetts, and Georgia, have enacted legislation requiring mental health coverage in any group health insurance plan. California has developed a legislative proposal which has a strong likelihood of enactment in 1973. In addition, California has made an effective presentation to the state insurance commissioner urging that state regulations require new group health plans to cover mental illness.

Costs of Mental Health Coverage

The APA report demonstrated that useful data are increasingly available with which to make judgments about the cost of insurance coverage of mental illness. Studies of outpatient treatment show that coverage of twenty sessions is enough in 90 percent of cases. The cost of such coverage is about $2.15 per individual per year. Short-term coverage for outpatient treatment is unquestionably feasible. The insurance carriers have been fearful of long-term re-educative psychotherapy and used psychoanalysis as a model of a type of treatment which could "break the plan." The suggestion that mental health professionals want to put every potential patient on a couch five times a week for five years each is obviously ridiculous. Few patients are suitable for analysis and still fewer analysts are available. This issue is raised repeatedly, however, and for this reason some positions suggest peer review at the end of twenty outpatient sessions. Furthermore, some suggest that long-term psychotherapy should be authorized only when there is loss of functioning and likelihood that hospitalization will be required. These kinds of limitations can be applied, but more to allay the fears of the carrier than because of any realistic experience.

The Reed Report also shows that inpatient treatment can be provided as well as inhospital treatment by a psychiatrist at a cost of less than 5 percent of the total benefits of any insurance plan. Indeed, it is clear that for a cost of four dollars per person per year a truly comprehensive series of mental health services can be covered and that a significant limitation is unnecessary. For chronic illness it is probably useful to have peer review in all instances (including mental health care).

Other data suggest that adequate coverage of mental illness would actually save money. A study of 256 patients of the Group Health Association in Washington, D.C., demonstrated that the use of psychiatric referral in the system produced a reduction in medical, surgical, and laboratory utilization of approximately 30 percent (Goldberg, Krantz, and Locke, 1970). A second study, which analyzed patients' use of mental health services under the Kaiser Foundation plan in 1960, also demonstrated that among patients receiving psychiatric benefits there was a "significant" reduction in the use of other medical services (Cumming and Follett, 1968).

HMO and CMHC

The community mental health center has evolved over the past decade. It provides comprehensive services, including prevention, to a geographic population. Funding has been from federal sources and matching funds from local and state resources as well as from patient fees. The health maintenance organization is receiving considerable attention and it will be an important part of the health care delivery system in the future. The HMO model often cited is the Kaiser-Permanente plan under which patients prepay (rather than paying a fee for service). Those served are a group of enrollees (rather than a geographic population). The services provided are for acute illness, although some services constituting true health maintenance may be included. Health maintenance organizations still wind up dealing predominantly with episodic illness. Emphasis on episodic acute care (as opposed to prevention) is one of the major criticisms of the HMO model.

In many areas explorations are under way to try to tie the community mental health center model to the HMO program. The HMO concept calls for a series of agreed upon services between the provider and the recipient. Enrollees must be persuaded that they need mental health coverage. In addition, providers must be persuaded that it is economically feasible to include this coverage. The Nixon Administration is hopeful that 90 percent of the people will be covered by an HMO arrangement by the end of this decade. The Administration position has also been that there is no incompatibility between the HMO concept and the CMHC concept. The HMO may well use the community mental health center as a contract agency to provide mental health services to its enrollees. Many feel that there is an advantage in having community mental health services *and* HMOs operating cooperatively.

Community Involvement in Mental Health

Many questioned how one can develop community accountability and responsibility. In view of NIMH interest in this area many wondered what kind of training would be required to establish delivery of mental health care by a variety of paraprofessionals and community workers. Developing community accountability and responsibility means involving medically trained people in an alien procedure. The key word here is education, and the process requires educating people in the community as well as the professionals.

Students must acquire new kinds of skills, including consultation to institutions whose approach to dealing with people is different from that of medical institutions.

People who control the organization and funding of mental health services are generally from the middle class. Some question the idea that those in control will truly be interested in disadvantaged populations. Psychiatry practiced in a ghetto situation is constantly related to funding and raises many deep issues among minority mental health professionals who are concerned about the misuse of traditional services. This concern is one of the driving forces behind the concept of community control. Minority professionals need to develop funding programs and institutions to meet existing needs. A delivery system which will not attend to the social problems of the ghetto is also a real source of distress to such communities.

Epilogue

Prospects for the Seventies

DONALD G. LANGSLEY

The sixties have featured widespread dissatisfaction with our health care system. "Health care is a right, not a privilege" is the slogan of all political parties and the main theme of a cry for reorganizing service delivery systems. Those who criticize point to the lack of health sciences manpower and to distribution of physicians and others in the healing professions who are concentrated in middle-class, urban-suburban areas. The poor, the minority groups, and those who live in rural areas lack the high quality of care familiar to those who live in the city. Criticism has also been leveled at the focus on treating diseases after they develop rather than on preventing them. Others decry the overemphasis on the most expensive professional groups and call for new team models which will make quality health care available to all citizens.

Recognizing the shortage of health professionals, many new medical schools have been developed. At the beginning of 1972 there were twenty-eight medical schools classified as "provisional" or "under development." Some had not yet admitted the first class. Others were about to grant their first group of M.D. degrees. It is particularly significant for health science educators that opportun-

147

ities for innovation and change are far greater in a new school than in an established one, where change threatens existing programs. Those who planned and started new medical schools were able to attract faculty with surprising ease, since the creative teacher recognized how unique the opportunity was.

Although there have been previous reforms in medical education, the reexamination represented in this book is occurring at a time when *traditional* is a pejorative term and when innovation is valued for its own sake. The rate of change is remarkable! Even the post-Flexner reforms required several decades, and that era was not without complications. The move from a guild type of training to the establishment of a firm scientific basis for practice brought medical education into the universities. The activities of the medical school teacher shifted away from a prominent commitment to (private) practice. The new medical educator devoted all his time to the medical school. Scientific advances resulted in specialization and subspecialization. The post-Sputnik emphasis on research combined with a high degree of government funding further elevated the status of the scientist. Research rather than patient care brought promotion to the academician, and research funds paid part of the cost of medical education.

The seventies will undoubtedly change this pattern. The cry of this decade is for more emphasis on human services. Research though still generously supported by government is developing a lower priority. The combination of emphasis on human services and the call for reorganization of the health care delivery system cannot help but influence the new medical schools.

One might also ask why the mental health professions (which certainly include nonphysicians) would limit themselves to medical school settings. The answer to this straw man is that of course they do not. Nevertheless, medical schools include the most experienced teachers in the health sciences. Though sometimes justifiably criticized for being overly conservative they have also been an important source of new knowledge and new approaches to practice. The medical school does not limit itself to training physicians; its students are in training for all the health professions. Some of the medical schools have pioneered innovative service delivery systems. The

medical schools generally have the expertise for careful evaluation of
the existing and innovative approaches to the prevention and treatment of mental disorder. Medical school departments of psychiatry
(or divisions of mental health, as some of the newer organizations
are named) consist of academicians from all mental health professions. It is reasonable to *hope* that advances in practice as well as in
science may come from medical schools—or (as many are called
nowadays) "health science centers."

These views formed the rationale for the Conference on
Mental Health Education in New Medical Schools. The challenge
of the seventies could be met in these thirty new schools. There was
every reason to establish a conference between members of their
psychiatry departments. The participants were joined by consultants,
whose position papers helped to define the major issues and stimulate
discussion and interaction. Using a workshop-conference format the
group was small enough to meet as a whole. Each major topic
occupied half a day. The position papers were distributed in advance
rather than read at the conference. The discussion was recorded in
the hope that the product would be useful to mental health educators in all settings. Many issues were highlighted by the discussion,
and although it is customary to plead that more questions than
answers arose, some answers were proposed. No one expected unanimity, but there were surprising areas of concurrence. The participants all demonstrated a high degree of enthusiasm, a commitment
to a problem-solving approach, and a willingness to consider new
solutions. An air of optimism was the general affect in spite of an
acknowledgement of serious problems to be resolved.

In this chapter I summarize the issues and present some of
the solutions suggested. The new schools are here portrayed in rather
broad strokes. Detailed program descriptions from each school are
given in Appendix A. These, too, were distributed prior to the
conference. So far as I know, they are the only source of reasonably
complete information about mental health training programs in the
new medical schools. These programs will surely change within a
few years, but meanwhile they represent the proposals of one group
of educators. The reader is invited to examine these programs de-

scriptions in some detail if he is a mental health educator. Some of the experiments are truly exciting.

Interdepartmental Curricula

The new medical schools recognize the danger of the traditional lock-step curriculum in which more attention is paid to structure than content. One problem of any educational venture is that it is often unresponsive to change in knowledge or practice; it is designed to perpetuate the existing disciplines through the "department" structure; one finds "time" for new content or new patterns of clinical practice only at the expense of existing programs, since no department wants to "give up its time." The new schools (they are developing training programs) have the opportunity to create a structure which will promote rather than inhibit change. Taking advantage of this opportunity, some have organized curriculum content along interdepartmental lines. In the basic sciences (perhaps more often than in the clinical departments) there are no courses with departmental names. The traditional courses labeled "anatomy," "biochemistry," and so on are replaced by interdepartmental courses in which a committee takes the responsibility for teaching a curriculum organized along functional lines. The committee generally includes representatives from several departments. In such schools (such as McMaster, California–Davis, Missouri–Kansas City) the basic science curriculum includes a course on molecular and cell biology, a course entitled Introduction to Clinical Medicine, and an organ system approach which integrates study of normal structure and function with the understanding of pathophysiology and the treatment of disease. The goal is to promote integration of knowledge rather than memorization of fragmented facts. Teaching is an attempt to impart basic principles and a problem-solving approach. While the traditional departments continue as organizations for recruitment and faculty development and contribute to those courses having an interdepartmental structure, the course committees are responsible for teaching. The new schools which have experimented with this structure find that it is more responsive to change. Although departments are reluctant to alter the emphasis and particularly, the number of hours devoted to their own material, committees have far less reluctance to shift the content of the course or the teaching methods. Since the chairmanship of the course committee rotates, no individual or group feels that a change is a personal defeat or diminution of status.

Interdepartmental courses also have the advantage of bringing about closer integration of clinical content and are more likely to enhance the professional student's motivation. They are more likely to bring a clinician into the basic science arena. The preprofessional student spends his time in laboratories and libraries looking forward to the day when he will have contact with a "live patient." Today's medical student comes to professional school with a high degree of interest in social problems and health care delivery systems. He often becomes impatient with an educational system which confines him to the laboratory for another two years. Early introduction to clinical medicine and early contact with clinical teachers enhance his desire to master basic science principles and force the faculty to make basic science "relevant." The same situation reminds the medical educator that his goal is to produce a generalist rather than a specialist in his own image. Medical school faculty from the basic science departments have often been accused of teaching medical students the same way they train their graduate students in their own disciplines. The same charge has been leveled at the faculty of the clinical departments, who have been accused of teaching from a narrow subspecialist point of view. Just as the committee structure brings faculty from various departments together (in a large medical school this is a unique accomplishment in itself) it influences practice as well as curriculum content.

In the clinical department the problems are somewhat different, and some of the new medical schools have retained departmental rather than general clerkships. Part of the reason for the departmental clerkship is the availability of clinical material. Departments control beds and clinics and are responsible for organizing clinical services. The specialized facilities required in hospitals apparently necessitate departmental structures. The specialty approach in clinical practice is very much a reality and the American public will continue to demand the advantage of specialists while calling for more effective organization of primary care. Consequently the new medical schools have maintained departmental clerkships,

Some have organized general clerkships which represent an introduction to a full-time clinical assignment. The general clerkship is often run by several departments or may be under the sponsorship of a department of family practice. In this clerkship the emphasis is on developing skills and general patient workup and an understanding of basic principles of treating the more common diseases.

Another change is the decreased number of required clinical clerkships. While the pattern of required clerkships in general surgery, general medicine, psychiatry, pediatrics, and obstetrics-gynecology continues, rotations through subspecialties in medicine or surgery are more likely to be elective. This change also permits more flexibility in clinical education. Once the principle has been established that the subspecialty does not have to have a block of time for the sake of status, the generalist disciplines can organize the content of the clinical experience more flexibly, changing emphases or rotation more easily than could be done with a long list of short rotations through subspecialties.

New Settings for Educational Programs

The training of mental health professionals and other health science personnel has traditionally been hospital-based, reflecting advances in medical science which have originated in laboratories and specialized facilities. The advantage of this system to the patient with a complex illness are obvious. The advantages to the medical school faculty member have been to keep him close to the hospital and his adjacent research labs. The impact on medical education, however, has been to highlight specialization and rare disease. The medical student has suffered from lack of contact with primary care physicians and ordinary disease. He gets his degree under the impression that the hospital is the proper place for treating most patients and that the office (like the ambulatory clinics of many university hospitals) is the place for follow-up visits. The past decade has seen serious questions raised about the usefulness of this model for organizing health care services. The university hospital as the only or major teaching facility continues the pattern of more emphasis on specialty than on primary care. The hospital, though very necessary for serious illness, is not the ideal locus for treating most patients.

In psychiatry the tendency toward ambulatory care and the avoidance of unnecessary hospitalization has been particularly prominent. A generation ago psychiatric care meant long-term hospitalization or private office treatment for the wealthy and healthy. Long-term hospitalization resulted in institutionalism, the enhancement of chronicity, and the disruption of families. The development of psychotropic drugs and new forms of individual and group therapy along with a community mental health orientation demonstrated that most patients who had previously been hospitalized could be treated in ambulatory settings.

Such changes in patterns of practice call for reexamination of the settings for educational programs. It is no longer appropriate for a resident in psychiatry, an intern in clinical psychology, or students in social work to spend *most* of their clinical experience in a hospital. A setting more closely approximating that in which the student will practice would seem more appropriate.

Medical schools have also responded to the call for greater involvement in health care delivery and for participation in developing new delivery systems. The future is likely to see more emphasis on health care teams, greater involvement in prevention, and a move toward comprehensive approaches which include neighborhood ambulatory services as well as community and regional health care centers for the more seriously ill.

A practical factor in the development of thiry new medical schools is the lack of funds for capital construction. The two decades after World War II saw large infusions of federal funds for construction of health facilities. These included Hill-Burton funds for community hospitals as well as other programs for the construction of health science facilities. A few of the new schools have some support from the final years of that era. Others have been caught with demands for more service while federal and state governments have fewer resources for health facilities construction. In part this reduction is the result of increased demands for government funding of higher education and other human services. In part it is due to the large expenditures for defense and the Viet Nam war.

The times require new settings for training mental health professionals. One pattern calls for medical schools to use community hospitals rather than to build university hospitals. The assumption is that community hospitals have patients, laboratories, and other facilities for high-quality patient care. Why not put students in such a setting? Medical schools respond that community hospitals are already being used for postgraduate education, for training many types of health sciences personnel, and even for some clinical experience for medical students. They point to the lack of full-time teachers and the fact that private practitioners cannot abandon their patients in order to spend their time teaching. The administrative complications of open and closed staffs and of medical school control over clinical programs which are used for teaching compound the problems. In addition, community hospitals rarely have physical facilities for conferences and other educational exercises. Another factor is the (sometimes not so subtle) concern of the private practitioner that medical school programs will interfere with his practice. The concerns are not only economic but also involve status and other emotional considerations. In spite of the complications, many of the new medical schools are determined to begin an M.D. program without a university hospital and have done the major part of their planning around the use of community hospitals. The results are not yet available, since those schools which do not own a hospital or at least have professional control over one not owned by the university are the newest schools. They have not yet had the opportunity to test the system and to report their experience.

The community mental health center model is one of the more interesting experiments in health care delivery. Starting with a commitment to provide comprehensive services to a population, it uses an interdisciplinary mental health team to provide a broad array of services designed to meet the needs of the patient rather than to suit the requirements of the staff. Presenting a balance of preventive as well as direct services and using paraprofessionals along with appropriate community participation in planning, it may represent an appropriate model for other health care experiments. When combined with other health care services, including public health, medical, and dental care, and when integrated with welfare agencies and other human services, it may be even more pertinent to the needs of people. However, the community mental health center as a medical school training setting has certain problems. Those problems are reviewed by Langsley (1972). Briefly, they include (1) commitment of the faculty and community; (2) control; (3) broad content of training; (4) decentralization in neighborhood settings; (5) uncertainty of identity in the multidisciplinary team; (6) funding the cost of training; (7) need for rearranging the reward system for teachers; (8) provision for continuing education; (9) complications associated with interdisciplinary training; (10) need for careful evaluation. In the California–Davis program the department of psychiatry has taken the responsibility for providing mental health services for an entire county of 640,000 people (five catchment areas). Two areas are served by contract agencies but the medical school faculty serve three catchment areas. The county mental health program is the principle teaching base for the Davis program. The student is trained by a mental health team consisting of professional staff or faculty members. Training is the responsibility of all of the three teams, which are interdisciplinary and responsible for training students from all mental health professions. The teams are organized to provide longitudinal contact with patients and continuity of care. The student in that program learns to simultaneously treat outpatients, inpatients, and crisis intervention cases and acquires skill in mental health consultation. The theoretical orientation is eclectic, and although prevention-consultation is valued, the faculty feel that one cannot be an effective community psychiatrist without being a skilled clinician. Each team has sufficient staff to treat all the patients, and students are assigned to the program for training, not service. Residents spend the first year with one catchment area mental health team and the second year with another team; the third year is elective.

California–Davis is only one of a number of new schools which made a commitment to a community mental health setting as a teaching base. Arizona, Michigan State, Missouri–Kansas City, New York–Stony Brook, Texas–San Antonio, and others have committed themselves to provide mental health services for a catchment area or part of one. Since the community mental health center focuses on ambulatory services, is often located away from an institutional setting, and offers a clear mixture of treatment modalities using an interdisciplinary team, this type of setting should be followed closely as one experiment in health sciences education.

Length of Training

The three-year medical curriculum has received considerable attention. It has been said that 30 percent of the M.D. graduates this year have completed a three-year course in medical school and that in two years 70 percent of the graduates will receive their M.D. in three calendar years. In part this reduction in length is the result of using the summer, so that medical school really consists of eleven or twelve academic quarters—not really a shortening of training (many programs only have three quarters per year) but a rearrangement of time.

The elimination of the internship requirement is proceeding rapidly; in another two or three years the internship as it was previously known will probably no longer exist. Here the motivation was to shorten training. The rationale is that medical students now have the same curriculum content and patient care experiences which used to belong to the internship. The senior year in most medical schools is really a rotating internship—often with much of the choice of clinical service being up to the student.

The members of the conference preferred to look at the overall educational program. The issue was not a shortening of medical school or the elimination of the internship but rather the total length of time from preprofessional training through completion of specialty training. Some members of experimental programs were interested in the length of time to award the M.D. degree. They often felt that three years of premedical education were sufficient and that four years of medical school could be compressed into three. Thus eight years could be reduced to six. Another experiment (Missouri–Kansas City) sought to combine premedical and medical education in a six-year course, taking students directly out of high school. The combination of a traditional premedical curriculum with early introduction to medical school itself is proving to be one of the most interesting experiments in the country.

Other educators were concerned with the length of time required to produce a specialist. In their schools the focus is on medical school plus specialty training and there, too, they are trying to reduce the number of years of formal education. Instead of four years of medical school, a year of internship, and at least three years of specialty training, some faculty feel that with three years of medical school, elimination of the internship, and the student going directly into a three-year specialty training program, a medical school could produce a specialist in six years instead of the traditional eight.

Some question the elimination of the internship and any reduction in the length of the medical curriculum. The pertinent questions cannot yet be answered because there is insufficient experience. Those schools which have had experience in taking M.D. graduates directly into a psychiatric residency without an internship are convinced that those first-year residents who had an internship are indistinguishable at the end of three to six months from the ones who did not. The selection process is cited as an important factor, and program directors generally concern themselves with the amount of patient care responsibility which the M.D. graduate (without internship) will have had. The program directors were also concerned about the degree of psychological maturity exhibited by the various applicants.

Other medical educators point to the need for flexibility in the length of the medical curriculum. Too few admissions committees or educators take into account the fact that people learn at different rates. For some who are fast learners and possessed of general maturity, six years may be sufficient. The curriculum planners also need to provide for the slow learner and for less mature individuals. They urge that more attention be paid to the individual student than to a rigid period of training. Others caution about the danger of premature career choice and remind us that people do change their minds after beginning a residency training program. Again, the more rational approach would be to individualize as much as possible and to carefully evaluate the results of experimental curricula which shorten the length of time in graduate school, medical school, or work in graduate education.

Minority Groups and Ethnic Subcultures

The new medical schools (as well as many of the established schools) are keenly aware of their responsibility to *all* citizens.

Medical educators are quite aware of the lack of health care for minority groups and for people who live in rural areas. This lack is reflected in serious health problems among those groups, including shorter life expectancy, a higher incidence of chronic disease, and significantly higher infant mortality rates. It is also a matter of concern that members of minority groups and the children of the poor do not have the same opportunities to obtain a medical education as do white, middle-class Americans. These problems point to two areas of need—providing health services for minority groups, and minority staff recruitment and minority student training.

Providing health care for minority groups and poor people is more complicated than merely training more physicians to work in poverty areas. Health care services for ethnic minorities must take cognizance of the environment and culture in which those individuals reside. Medical students and other mental health professionals must be instructed in the social and cultural backgrounds and needs of minorities. In these times a condescending approach of charity care will not do. Citizens from all groups deserve to have high-quality care offered in a respectful and humane manner which will be realized in such a way that it will be used by the citizens who need it.

Minority staff recruitment is essential, and most schools have undertaken an affirmative action program. The staffs of medical schools and health care agencies need to be representative of the entire population. Students should learn about minority subcultures from minority individuals themselves. This requisite has placed a special strain on the obviously limited number of minority health professionals. Those schools engaged in an affirmative action program must make extra effort to recruit minority faculty and staff and yet maintain the highest possible quality of health care and health sciences educational programs.

And finally, the times call for more minority students. Here, too, recruitment problems are not simple. Minority students are often educationally disadvantaged. To expect them to meet the same academic criteria as white, middle-class students is unrealistic. To graduate second-class doctors is equally unrealistic. Admissions committees must try to identify those who have the potential for completing educational programs in medicine or other health science professions and to make the special effort required to recruit such students and to bring them through the curriculum successfully. Not a small task! The new schools are highly motivated in this area. Yet they often lack the financial resources of the established schools. Finding support for such programs is an important challenge for the seventies.

Behavioral Sciences

The basic behavioral sciences have traditionally been part of the curriculum of the departments of psychiatry. A number of departments have sections or divisions of behavioral sciences; others do not have a separate administrative entity but appoint basic scientists to the regular faculty of the department. Still others borrow staff from existing departments whose disciplines are relevant to understanding human behavior. For the most part these have been the social behavioral sciences (sociology, anthropology, social psychology), but there is now a tendency to include the more biologically oriented behaviorists, such as neurophysiologists and experimental psychologists. A few schools have experimented with a separate department of behavioral sciences in the hope that a new discipline of basic behavioral sciences can evolve. In fact these experiments are very controversial. The departments of psychiatry in the four or five schools which have a separate department of behavioral science are not at all pleased with the results. In spite of the provocative position paper by Resnik, almost all the psychiatrists at the conference responded negatively. They point to the fact that the behavioral sciences are not a single discipline but a conglomerate of disciplines. Ask a faculty member in a department of behavioral science what he is and he will tell you that he is an anthropologist or a social psychologist or a neurophysiologist. He will not respond "I am a behavioral scientist." There seems to be no special reason why individuals from varying disciplines will have an easier time of collaborative teaching or cooperative research in a separate department than they would have in a department of psychiatry. Generally such individuals are research-oriented and have no clinical responsibility and do little teaching. At this stage of development, and in the present context of limited resources for developing new medical schools, it may be more sensible to maintain the dialogue between clinicians and behavioral scientists by housing them in the same departments. The behavioral sciences have not yet achieved a level of development where research on human behavior is easily quantified or become a single discipline, such as biochemistry or physiology. The problems are not likely to be solved by creating a separate department.

Funding Services and Training

Money is no small problem for the new medical schools. As a matter of fact, money is a serious problem for the health sciences in general. As has been noted previously, the demand for vastly increased amounts of health services comes at a time when unlimited funds are not available to pay for them. The cost of health care—especially hospital services—rises in an almost uncontrolled fashion. High-quality health care is never going to be cheap; neither is high-quality education for health professionals.

When services are more expensive and funds are less available the third-party funding agencies such as insurance plans and government are no longer willing to have graduate medical education piggybacked on the cost of hospitalization. The fact that research funds are less readily available will diminish the extent to which medical education is supported by research. Medical education is getting squeezed in the crunch, and a number of medical schools have been in serious economic difficulty. Recent federal capitation schemes offer bonuses for increasing the size of a class, but the awards do not pay the full cost of the educational programs. It is likely that the government will consider this "seed money" instead of permanent commitment to fund all the costs of medical education.

Medical schools will clearly have to be more concerned with health care delivery. While it is not realistic to suggest that medical education can be supported by the clinical work of the faculties, it is equally unrealistic to deny that clinical programs spin off an educational benefit.

In addition to experiencing economic pressures, medical schools are also being pressed to devise and demonstrate new approaches to health care delivery. They cannot deny their responsibilities for innovation and evaluation. A number of the HMO experiments have been associated with medical schools. The school obviously has the manpower resources to experiment in this area as well as the research expertise to evaluate the results. At the same time the medical school must be sure that its efforts in this direction are consonant with its primary mission—education and research. The balance between service, teaching, and research is undoubtedly shifting somewhat in the direction of increased emphasis on service. That shift must not destroy the training program or the next generations will suffer seriously.

In the field of psychiatry and the other mental health professions this problem is especially complex. Most third-party payment plans have poor coverage for mental illness or do not cover it at all. The government has traditionally assumed responsibility for mental illness by paying for the cost of state hospital care. Only recently has it become apparent that treating mental illness in the community is less expensive than using the state hospital model. The benefits have not yet caught up, however. Under most insurance programs, benefits for inpatient care are far more generous than for ambulatory treatment. Some treatment approaches such as partial hospitalization are labeled as "not treatment at all but only room and board." Third-party payers do not cover preventive services or mental health consultation to agencies.

At the federal level a number of proposals have been made for a national health insurance scheme. Although a comprehensive national health insurance program will probably not be enacted within the year is it not many years away. The intermediate model may well be the health maintenance organization, which is committed to providing the full range of direct services to a preenrolled population on a prepaid basis. The population is generally not geographic but rather the number of individuals who have enrolled in a plan. But the HMOs that have been developed offer minimal benefits for psychiatric illness. Of the first 106 HMOs only eight have any mental health treatment benefits at all. The suggestion that the HMO model will replace the community mental health center model is not a solution. The community mental health center with its commitment to a geographic population and its funding of preventive services has advantages not available in the HMO. The mental health professions will really need both models while some national health insurance scheme is being worked out. The mental health professions will have to be especially careful to see that mental illness and mental disorder have adequate coverage. If not, then the one in ten who needs treatment for such disorder at some time during his life will be deprived.

Conclusion

One can only conclude that the seventies will indeed present serious challenges for mental health educators. The new schools and the other settings in which mental health training programs are carried on will have to attend closely to the experiments in curriculum development—particularly the interdepartmental and interdisciplinary approaches. Training programs will surely be carried on in untraditional settings. The experiments with the organization of graduate and postgraduate training in the mental health professions will necessitate careful evaluation and varied models of individualized programs and different track systems. Affirmative action recruiting and special attention to health services for minority groups require constant monitoring. The mental health professionals who wanted to ignore the realities of funding will certainly not be able to do so; indeed they must become leaders in solving economic problems. And finally, with reexamination and recertification just around the corner, programs of continuing education must help keep the practitioner abreast of new developments.

There is no lack of challenge for the seventies! The new schools have the vigor and opportunity to help meet those challenges.

Program Descriptions of Mental Health Education in the New Medical Schools

ⵣⵣⵣⵣⵣⵣⵣⵣⵣⵣⵣⵣⵣⵣⵣⵣⵣⵣⵣⵣⵣⵣⵣⵣⵣ

University of Arizona

Since its inception the basic operating philosophy of the Department of Psychiatry in regard to its teaching program has focused on two points. One of these is the development of teaching activities in close collaboration with the other clinical services of the College of Medicine. This plan has been implemented by establishing teaching activities not only within psychiatric inpatient and out-patient settings but also within clinic and hospital services operated by the Department of Internal Medicine, the Department of Obstetrics and Gynecology, and the Department of Pediatrics. The second major element in the Department of Psychiatry's basic philosophy is a commitment to a primary emphasis on teaching clinical skills, with a corollary emphasis on teaching how to apply these skills in the many different types of settings in which psychiatry is now practiced. This commitment is being implemented through

163

the development of teaching activities not only in the inpatient unit and clinic of the Arizona Medical Center, but also in a community mental health program, a private psychiatric hospital, and a county facility.

At the present time, the principal clinical teaching for medical students is provided by the Department of Psychiatry during the third year. During this year each student has a six-week clinical clerkship in psychiatry, and during this time he is assigned primarily to an inpatient psychiatric setting. The Department of Psychiatry is also responsible for teaching in the other three years of the current medical school curriculum. During the first year, the department offers a course which is designed to be a basic introduction to behaviorial science generally and to provide also specialized instruction in such areas as human development and human sexuality. During the second year, each student takes the department's lecture course, which introduces psychopathology and clinical diagnosis. The second-year curriculum also includes specialized instruction by the Department of Psychiatry in interviewing techniques and the process of the mental status examination. At the present time, the College of Medicine curriculum for the fourth year provides for a series of elective experiences, and the Department of Psychiatry offers fourth-year students a variety of clinical electives.

The faculty of the College of Medicine has recently voted to endorse a new curriculum which will enable students to receive their medical degree after three years. This new curriculum involves thirty-three months of instruction and three months of vacation during the three-year period. Under the proposed new curriculum, the Department of Psychiatry will have the same kinds of responsibilities that it has now. The basic behavioral science and human development instruction will be provided during the first year, the introductory clinical material will be presented early in the second year, and the clinical clerkship will continue to be one of the clinical courses required of all students.

Brown University

In 1963, Brown University launched a program in medical education based on the challenging concept of integrating medical education within the fabric of a university. Taking advantage of existing strength in the physical and biological sciences, Brown elected to develop a six-year continuum merging the usual college experience with the first two years of a standard medical school. The primary objective was "to prepare medical scientists and physicians who are capable of future leadership in academic medicine, research, and clinical practice."

The concept of the physician-scholar remains as valid now as it was when the first Brown faculty committee defined it ten years ago. The challenge for us is to accept the duality of medicine, with its foundation in the natural and social sciences and its focus on the human being in distress. We must go beyond superficial distinctions between medical research and medical practice, the health care value of specialists versus generalists. We must retain and expand scholarship and at the same time be adaptable and responsive to the needs of our students and of society in general. If we fail, we will find ourselves in a quiet backwater, a relatively unimportant force in graduate education. If we succeed, we may provide a model of interdisciplinary education while demonstrating that we care for the community of which Brown is a part.

Our goals are: to operate not a traditional medical school but an educational program within the university with recognizable academic characteristics and provision of a limited number of parallel tracks toward the M.D. degree not usually available in medical schools; to make this program the hub of the Rhode Island health education and health care delivery system, and as such to welcome participation of all interested institutions (colleges and hospitals); to help in the development and coordination of state-wide plans for health care delivery at an acceptable cost; to help in the expansion of a health-related industry in Rhode Island.

The curriculum envisioned for the Brown model for specialty training is an extension of the current six-year program, leaving the first five years essentially unchanged, substituting a rotation of clerkship for the current sixth year, and including in the seventh year part of what is currently the internship experience. After 1975, the student is expected to enter the first year of a residency program immediately after obtaining his M.D. degree; thus the proposed curriculum eliminates two years from the current course of studies from high school graduation to residency (seven instead of nine years). Student participation, however, is anticipated on the basis of eleven months per year starting in the summer following the third year.

For convenience of exposition, this program is described in three blocks: the first three years; the intermediate two; and the last two years. Each summer period is appended to the following academic year. The description of course content is not intended as a rigid model but as an example and a basis for planning.

Block I. Year I—two courses in calculus, two courses in chemistry (physical and organic), one or two courses in biology (introductory), two courses at least in humanities or social sciences.

Year II—summer: free (experience suggests that a number of students will elect to conduct an independent study, to participate in a laboratory program, or to obtain a hospital experience). Academic year: one course in mathematics or applied mathematics (differential equations, computer programming); two courses in chemistry (organic and physical); two courses in physics (mechanics and electricity); one or two courses in biology (comparative anatomy, development, genetics), two courses in humanities, social, or behavioral Sciences.

Year III—summer: free (for some students at least, same experience as during the previous summer, either in the United States or abroad). Academic year: three to four courses in biomedical sciences (introductory biochemistry, molecular biology and molecular genetics; cell physiology and biophysics, and histology-embryology). One course in psychology (experimental), one course in sociology (medical), possibly a course in applied mathematics (computer programming) or physics (such as electronics or modern physics), two courses in the humanities or social Sciences. Examination: MCAT (Medical College Admission Test) in October or May.

First Checkpoint. Following completion of the first three years in the program, the student may elect to continue as a regular senior in the college (and apply to medical school if he so desires) or apply for continuation in the Medical Science Program. In the latter case, a check of his ability, performance, and motivation will be made on the basis of his academic performance (minimum of twenty-four course credits), MCAT score, career motivation, and deree of fit with characteristics of the program, as determined by an interview and a study of his record.

Block II. Year IV—summer: (optional) one or two courses in research in a clinical, experimental, or health-related setting. Possibly one independent study in any field. Academic year: five courses in biomedical science (human anatomy, systems physiology, pharmacology, general pathology, microbiology, immunology), one or two courses in behavioral science, clinical psychology, and introductory psychiatry, one or two other courses in humanities or social sciences. Degree: B.A. or B.S. on completion of requirements for any specific undergraduate concentration. Checkpoint: Transfer to graduate school based on appropriate performance in year IV and receipt of a bachelor's degree.

Year V—summer: one course in physical diagnosis in a clinical setting; one course in research. Academic year: a year-long course (two credits) in neurosciences, including neuroanatomy, neurophysiology, neuropharmacology, and neuropathology. Two year-long courses in organ-system pathophysiology (cardiovascular, respiratory, renal, and blood first semester; gastroenterology, endocrinology, and growth and development in the second semester). Two courses in humanities or social studies. Examination: National Board of Medical Examiners Part I in June of fifth year. Degree: Master of Medical Science upon completion of graduate school requirements (eight courses at graduate level in area of concentration—no more than two of which are in research—and presentation and acceptance of a thesis).

Second Checkpoint. Following completion of the first five years (or equivalent) the student has the option to transfer to another medical school in advanced standing or to apply for continuation at Brown. In the latter case, a formal review will be conducted stressing adequate performance in years IV and V of the program, demonstration of interest and ability in patient care, and passing Part I of the National Board, but not requiring completion of M.M.S. thesis.

Block III. Year VI—the twelve-month period starting July 1 will be divided into three periods, one of three months (July-September) and two or four months (October-January, and February-

May). Each of these periods will be devoted to a clinical clerkship, two of which will be hospital-based ("medicine" and "surgery") and one based in ambulatory care centers ("community medicine"). The student may elect to postpone the summer clerkship to the following summer in order to complete his master's thesis. The clerkships may be arranged to permit students to take one elective course per semester during the same period, that is, up to three over the twelve-month period.

Year VII—the summer is devoted to one of the clinical clerkships if necessary, or to completion of a research project, or to independent study. The academic year is divided into two periods corresponding to the academic semesters. Students spend one of these periods in elective activities (campus, hospital, or elsewhere) and one in a full-time internship experience. Examination: National Board Part II must be taken in June of the seventh year. Degree: the M.D. degree is awarded at the end of the seventh year.

University of Connecticut

Medical Student Education: First and Second Years. The first two years of the combined medical-dental basic science program consist of sequential Interdisciplinary Teaching Committees to which all students devote their full time. All departments work together in the development, teaching, supervision, and evaluation of all subject committees. The initial half of the first year is devoted to cell, tissue, and pathological biology as these apply to all organ systems, and to the social and behavioral science basis of clinical medicine and dentistry. The second half of the first year, and nearly all of the second year, involves study of the organ systems, in sequence and in a manner which permits detailed consideration of each system. Material from microbiology, pathology, pharmacology, and the clinical disciplines is studied as each organ system is discussed.

The Social and Behavioral Sciences Subject Committee is the first teaching committee for first-year students. The Department of Psychiatry presents twenty-five of the eighty-four hours in this committee, focusing on individual development, family structure and dynamics, the life-history method, and interviewing technique. During this subject committee, extensive use is made of audio-visual aides, such as commercial films illustrating the dynamics of personality development and family interaction and videotaped life-history interviews of psychiatric patients.

Within this committee, each student elects to spend fifteen hours of concentrated study in seminar sessions on one of the following areas: (1) poverty, ethnicity, and health, (2) social welfare, (3) community health action program, (4) theories and methods of change in health practice, (5) identity formation—Erikson's psychosocial formulations, and (6) issues in the establishment of a national health service.

The Department of Psychiatry also provides extensive input into the 190-hour Central Nervous System Subject Committee, with a total of twenty-three classroom hours and twenty-four psychiatry laboratory hours. Our focus in this committee is on psychiatric interviewing; defense mechanisms; correlative physiological, chemical and epidemiological data; psychopathologic states; and theories relevant to the etiology and pathogenesis of mental disease. Students are assisted in developing an ability to differentiate psychopathologic symptoms through use of the SAID (Systems Analysis Index for Diagnosis of Basic Psychiatric Syndromes) handbook.

Under the Central Nervous System Subject Committee, the Department of Psychiatry offers two elective laboratories in which the student investigates a hypothesis relating social factors to psychopathology or to psychotherapeutic drug effects. These laboratories are conducted in sixteen hours spaced over four weeks. The CNS laboratories acquaint the students with research design, statistical analysis of data, and interpretation and presentation of results.

Psychiatry is integrated with other medical specialties in teaching the Introduction to Clinical Medicine, with 280 hours of direct patient contact over the first two years; psychiatry's input is thirty-two hours in the first and second years.

The fourth committee in which the Department of Psychiatry plays a major role is the Growth and Development Committee, the final course of the second year. The twenty full-class hours of psychiatric teaching cover psychological and social development, family and intergenerational dynamics, adolescence, mental health of the poor, abortion, suicide, aging, and death. Individual, interpersonal, and sociocultural processes are explored in depth. The concurrent Introduction to Clinical Medicine provides an opportunity for the practical application and integration of theoretical material presented in Growth and Development and previous committees.

In addition to these areas of major participation in teaching committees, selected psychiatry input is included in the Endocrine and Reproductive System and Gastrointestinal System Subject Committees during the second year. In the Endocrine and Reproductive System Committee, material is presented on human sexuality, gender identity, gender assignment, and the modern treatment of human sexual inadequacy: a total of four full-class sessions, with related elective experiences for interested students.

In the Gastrointestinal Committee the Department of Psychiatry organizes didactic material on hunger and obesity, peptic ulcer, gastric secretion and psychic states, and colitis. A laboratory experience is also provided, presenting the students with a psychosomatic disease model. In this laboratory, the physiological, social, and psychological data obtained by the medical students from interviewing and performing lab tests on patients with either duodenal ulcer or lower gastrointestinal tract disease and from normal controls are integrated and tested statistically.

The final area of Department of Psychiatry involvement in the first two years of medical/dental education is in the credit elective program, offered to both first- and second-year students. The psychiatric elective is a 108-hour seminar on Human Sexual Behavior. Aimed at increasing general knowledge and desensitizing the students' personal reactions to sexual behavior, information provided by this course will enable the students to recognize sexual problems and to deal effectively with people with sexual disorders.

Medical Student Education: Third and Fourth Years. The Introductory Clerkship is the first concentrated clinical learning experience of third-year medical students and is a twelve-week rotation through medicine, pediatrics, and psychiatry. Six weeks are devoted to inpatient services of the three specialties; the second six-week segment is devoted to outpatient services of the three specialties. The clerkship is planned and presented by faculty of the three departments principally concerned, who also serve as preceptors for the students for close supervision of their clinical experience. The clinical experience is correlated with didactic sessions on interviewing techniques, major diagnostic categories, differential diagnosis and case management.

The Selective Clerkship in Psychiatry is a one- or two-month clinical experience in both inpatient and outpatient care. In addition to receiving supervision of their day-to-day clinical work, students participate in the following weekly programs: three ninety-minute sessions on psychiatric theory, a ninety-minute series on interviewing technique, professor's rounds, and case conference. The series on psychiatric theory includes specific diagnostic syndromes, personality development, defense mechanisms, dreams, psychotherapy, psychosomatic medicine, psychological testing, social psychiatry, child psychiatry, preventive and community psychiatry, and forensic psychiatry.

Residency Training. The University of Connecticut Department of Psychiatry will have eighteen residents in training when the program reaches full strength. The Residency Training Program emphasizes continuity of patient care between community and hospital with a deemphasis of divison between inpatient, outpatient, and emergency treatment facilities. The clinical experience of each resident incorporates supervised responsibilities in each of these areas through his assignment with appropriate treatment teams. This program emphasizes preparation for community-based service and academic psychiatry over private practice.

The first year of the program emphasizes the principles of normal child development, the treatment of childhood disorders, and community-based outpatient psychiatric experiences. The second year is based on the inpatient services. In this way the resident has the opportunity to have an experience with normal development and less severe psychopathology before being introduced to more seriously disturbed hospitalized patients. In addition, he brings to the hospital year of his training the experience of working with community agencies and a knowledge of the resources available there for the more complete care of his patient.

During the entire twelve months the first year the resident spends three half days a week in one of the affiliated child psychiatry programs. A variety of clinical work with children, including individual psychotherapy (short- and long-term), family therapy, and clinical supervision, is coordinated with formal didactic sessions on personality deviation, psychopathology, and personality development.

From September to June a fourth half day is spent in consultation to schools or the police regarding children's problems. Of the remaining three days of the resident's time, two are devoted to community-based outpatient experiences and one to didactic material. The community experience is presently built around the Crisis Intervention Unit (CIU). Residents make home visits as part of a team that includes a social worker and a nurse. They also consult with community agencies and do short-term family therapy and other short-term interventions.

First-year residents begin to do individual adult psychotherapy under supervision in August and September. They also serve as consultants to the other clinical departments concerning the latter's patients with psychiatric problems. As a part of their liaison service experience the residents are also assigned to the Psychosomatic Clinic, where they see medical outpatients under supervision.

The didactic program consists initially of a core curriculum taught during the first year of residency. This core curriculum will lead into four tracks: biobehavioral; intrapsychic personality dynamics; sociointerpersonal; and sociocultural. Department of Psychiatry faculty and clinical associates conduct sessions on history-taking and mental status examination, psychiatric syndromes, principles and practices of disciplines associated with psychiatry, psychological testing, group therapy, research methodology, the history of psychiatry, nonverbal communication, and theoretical psychiatry.

Teaching for each of the four tracks begins in the second year. The second- and third-year didactic program consists principally of research seminars or reviews of actual research programs under way in each of the track areas; advanced therapeutic application seminars; and seminars directed at the integration of the four tracks.

The clinical program for the second year of residency training is primarily based on the inpatient services of affiliated community hospitals. The second-year resident is directly involved in evaluating the potential admission to the inpatient service from the emergency room and the community. The same resident completes the collection of data, diagnostic evaluation, and formulation of a treatment plan for all patients admitted by him. He coordinates his treatment interventions with the other members of his treatment team at regularly scheduled meetings.

The resident continues to manage his patients after discharge from the hospital in the team follow-up clinic. There are separate interdisciplinary teams in the community-services outpatient unit similar to those in the inpatient unit. Though the second-year resident is primarily based on inpatient service, he maintains continuity of care of his patients, sees potential admissions in a nonhospital setting during a crisis situation, and gains continued experience in using community resources to help manage his patients. In addition, under supervision he continues to treat outpatients who have never been hospitalized.

The third-year program is devoted to elective time. Residents choose to deepen their educational and clinical experiences in areas that are of particular interest to them. The majority of third-year residents elect a clinical base for their year. On a clinical service they are responsible for supervision of junior residents and trainees from other disciplines. The residents also assume some responsibility for teaching medical students and nonpsychiatric house officers who are assigned to their clinical unit.

University of California–Davis

The Division of Mental Health (Department of Psychiatry), following the pattern of the entire medical school, has developed educational and clinical programs with like rapidity. In a fashion most unusual for a medical school, it has accepted the responsibility for mental health services for an entire county of 650,000 people. The chairman of the Department of Psychiatry is also director of Mental Health Services for Sacramento County. The professional staff of the Sacramento County Mental Health Service is the major part of the full-time faculty of the Department of Psychiatry and has been recruited by the School of Medicine. Three generic catchment area teams have become the interdisciplinary teachers of medical students, psychiatric residents, clinical psychologists, social workers, nurses, and other groups. A child psychiatry training program and a Ph.D. program in community-clinical psychology began in 1972. The clinical program has dramatically reduced the utilization of state hospital services. Emphasis on crisis intervention has further reduced the use of hospitalization within the community. Children's services are of high priority and integrated with adult treatment programs. Special attention has been given to minority groups, drug abuse, and alcoholism problems. From a central hospital base, multiservice neighborhood health centers have been developed.

The particular focus of this division is that educational programs are carried on with a special commitment to the delivery of mental health services. *Training is truly interdisciplinary and is carried on in the realistic setting of a mental health team. There is continuity of educational experience for the student and continuity of clinical treatment for the patient.*

Medical Student Education. The medical-student curriculum features integrated rather than departmental teaching and early clinical experience, and half of the curriculum is available for electives. The student attends school for fifteen consecutive quarters after matriculation. The first and second years of core curriculum include twenty hours a week of instruction, and in the third year there are full-time clinical clerkships. The fourth year is entirely elective. In the first year there are four courses: Molecular and Cell Biology; Organ and System Biology; Behavioral Biology; and Clinical Medicine. Psychiatry faculty teach in two of the four courses and provide 80 percent of the instructional time in Behavioral Biology and 40 percent of the instructional time in Clinical Medicine (interviewing, history-taking, and physical diagnosis). Behavioral Biology focuses on the biopsychosocial determinants of behavior from a developmental point of view and includes instruction on culture, poverty, and relevant information on health care delivery systems. In the sophomore year the curriculum is divided into nine organ systems. Psychiatry faculty teach in six of these organ systems and provide a major block of instruction on disorders of behavior using the multimedia SAID program. This program, developed by Miller and Tupin at Davis, is now being used at eighteen other medical schools. In the junior year the student has twelve required weeks of medicine, twelve of surgery, twelve of maternal-child health, six of psychiatry, and six weeks of clinical electives. Junior medical students serve their psychiatric clerkship on a community mental health team and on the crisis service. The goal of the instruction is to focus on those types of problems which the nonpsychiatric physician is most likely to encounter and to have to manage himself. A student is required to treat patients (under supervision) as the person responsible for that patient. His teachers include representatives from all the mental health professions. The Department of Psychiatry has also developed nineteen elective courses, including a research seminar on family psychology, courses on the sociology of mental illness, family and marital counseling, psychosomatic problems, and medical aspects of human sexuality. In addition there are full-time clinical electives which provide instruction on mental health teams, in neighborhood mental health centers, and in child psychiatry services on mental health teams; pediatric liaison experience; instruction on the child in trouble, drug abuse, crisis intervention, and antisocial behavior; outpatient psychotherapy; and off-campus clinical electives. The first medical student class taking Part II of the National Boards at the end of their third (rather than fourth) year averaged .2 percent above the national average in the five other clinical specialties and 2.2 percent above the national average in psychiatry.

Residency Training. The Department is conducting a three-year residency program in psychiatry carried on in a community mental health center. Training is oriented to produce generalists. The program is interdisciplinary, and all mental health professionals are trained in the same clinical setting. Child and adult services are integrated. The program is community-oriented with a balance of emphasis including individual psychotherapy and the other psychological and somatic therapies. Both indirect and direct services are part of the training program. The program consists of two years of required assignments and a third year of elective assignments. Each of the first two years consists of an assignment to one of the three community mental health teams of the Sacramento County Mental Health Service.

First year—a full-year assignment to a community mental health team. The team is responsible for the training and for all of the clinical work. The resident simultaneously treats inpatients, outpatients, and partial hospitalization patients, but there are more inpatient cases in the first year than the second. During this year the resident also has clinical experience on the Emergency/Crisis Service. He sees children as well as adults. He attends certain required seminars (three to five hours per week) and has three to five hours per week of individual supervision.

Second year—the second year is another full-year assignment to a different community mental health team. The format is similar to that of the first year except there is more emphasis on outpatient treatment, crisis intervention, and mental health consultation. The resident continues to treat any of his patients as outpatients or inpatients, as required. There is an assignment of six hours per week for six months to the Pediatric and Medical Psychiatric Liaison Service and four hours per week for nine months to the UCD Student Health Service. The resident attends three to four hours per week of required seminars and has two to three hours per week of individual supervision.

Third year—the third year is an elective year in which the resident may choose from a number of opportunities for broadening his skills. The possibilities include research opportunities, a state mental hospital, a forensic psychiatry setting, selected child psychiatry programs, an alcoholism program, or selected experiences with the Mental Health Service.

The department had in 1972–1973 ten first-year, seven second-year, and three third-year residents (on affiliation). There were 180 applications for the ten available residency positions.

Child Psychiatry Residency Training. The child psychiatry training program is based in the community mental health service, where child psychiatry services are integrated with the basic psychiatric services. The program trains child psychiatrists who are broadly based, experienced in community mental health techniques, competent in pediatric liaison services, and cognizant of the need for creating and extending relevant health care services beyond the confines of the hospital and mental health center. Trainees are provided closely supervised interdisciplinary experiences in a wide spectrum of psychodiagnostics, psychotherapy, pharmacotherapy, counseling, and collaboration, in a variety of health care and community facilities, including the developing child advocacy system. The fellow in child psychiatry works with minority groups and learns skills relative to the treatment and prevention of problems of youth in areas of drug abuse, delinquency, and sexual problems. Trainees teach and supervise medical students, pediatric and general psychiatry residents, and other mental health professionals as well as preprofessionals.

Other Educational Programs. Training for all the mental health professions occurs in the community mental health setting. The department is responsible for its own clinical psychology internship and presently has three interns. A Ph.D. in community-clinical psychology will be offered by the Division of Mental Health. Psychiatric social work students from Sacramento State College and psychiatric nursing students from Sacramento State College receive clinical training in the department (ten social work students and thirty-nine nursing students). The department also provides an internship in clinical pastoral counseling (six students), clinical experience for a human services program at American River College (ten students), and clinical experience for undergraduate college students (ten such). The medical psychiatric liaison program provides training in psychological problems of physical disease for house staff in the other medical specialties and for medical students on those nonpsychiatric specialty services. The efforts of almost two full-time faculty equivalents are devoted to this type of educational program. The program has had special success in medicine, pediatrics, and family practice. Three of the six faculty child psychiatrists are Board eligible or certified in pediatrics and hold appointments in both departments. Pediatric residents rotate on Child Psychiatry for two months.

Charles R. Drew Postgraduate Medical School

The Drew School will pursue health as a societal goal rather than treat disease as recurring crisis. Its mandate is to engage the unwieldy tools of a medical center to uplift the spirit and life style of a community as part of that community's health aspirations. The Drew School will adapt the traditional priorities of education, patient care, and research to serve the foremost needs of the community. This is not, we maintain, incompatible with the mission of the university and its obligations to society. We have been successful in recruiting the brightest and most resourceful academician-practitioners and we will continue our recruiting in that tradition. We are hopeful that the residents of Watts and its surrounding environment including all ethnic and cultural origins will be able to discern something of themselves in the Drew School and to recognize it as an instrument of healing and reconciliation and a focus of community pride.

The assumption of its social responsibilities does not diminish the school's obligations to create and advance knowledge. The unique duality of Drew's mission is that its research and educational endeavors will be valid only insofar as they buttress the School's societal goals. The implications of this "restructing" of the usual mission of an academic health institution are several. For example, in patient care, the efforts of the school will be directed toward ascertaining the real health needs of the community, identifying gaps in available services, and ultimately providing leadership in designing and helping to effect an organized system or network for providing the full range of comprehensive health care services to the community population which comprises approximately five hundred thousand persons, predominantly black, in a forty-square–mile area.

The University of South Florida

The College of Medicine was authorized by the state legislature in 1965. During the next three years, the university conducted an in-depth study relative to the site, cost, and possible programs for the new college. The first full-time dean of the College of Medicine was appointed in October 1969, and since that time plans have proceeded for physical facilities, curriculum, and recruitment of the medical faculty. The College of Medicine opened with the charter class in September 1971.

Throughout the period of development, the objectives of the college have remained foremost. First, we are seeking to create an academic environment in which medical education, the production of new knowledge, and community service may be conducted in a quality manner. Second, the College of Medicine is to be integrated into the mainstream of its community, will participate and lead in upgrading and improving the health care standards of the community in which the college is located. Third, the college is to function within the framework of the total university as an integral and valued part of the university community of scholars and students.

With these concepts in mind, a curriculum has been developed to accomplish these goals. The medical student will be introduced to clinical medicine in the first year, beginning with a period devoted exclusively to clinical orientation, followed by clinical correlation conferences continuing throughout the entire year. Although study in the basic sciences is concentrated in the first year, such education will be continued throughout the entire curriculum; for example, a basic science review is included in each clinical clerkship, and a generous amount of elective time provided for the final year permits electives to be chosen in the basic science areas at the discretion of the student and his advisors. Clinicians will participate in all basic science courses and generous use will be made of the basic scientists throughout the clinical work.

Beginning with the class entering in July of 1972, a three-year program will be followed. This pattern aims to substitute a thirty-three–month total curricular program achieved in three years for the thirty-six–month pattern followed in the traditional four-year schedule. This goal will be accomplished by continuing instruction throughout the calendar year with only brief vacations at appropriate breaks in the program. The assignments of time have been arranged in blocks so that for special reasons or under particular circumstances, a given student might extend his time beyond the scheduled three-year pattern, at the discretion of the faculty.

First Year. Students will devote their major activities to the basic medical sciences throughout this year. The purpose of these courses is to teach principles rather than an array of unrelated facts. Relevance to medicine is emphasized in all areas of instruction. Following a period of clinical orientation, students will be introduced to anatomy, biochemistry, physiology, medical microbiology, pathology and laboratory medicine, and pharmacology. This year will also include introductory courses in medicine and physical diagnosis and in behavioral sciences as well as introductory tutorial clerkships preparatory to the standard clerkship pattern to be followed in the succeeding year.

Second Year. This entire year will be devoted to clinical clerkships with basic science reviews included within each. Clerkships will be assigned in medicine, surgery, pediatrics, obstetrics, gynecology, and psychiatry.

Third Year. This year will be entirely elective. The program is set up so as to permit one twenty-week elective or two ten-week electives in each half of this academic year. Provision has been made for an eighty-hour elective review as the final exercise immediately preceding graduation. Choice of electives will be governed by the particular interests and needs of individual students and may be in either clinical fields or basic science. Off-campus work at other medical centers will be permitted under suitable direction and with the advice of the faculty. Opportunities will also be offered during this final year for students' participation in research with faculty and for in-depth clinical tutorial assignments as designed and indicated.

The Department of Psychiatry, established in September 1970, was the first clinical department created in the College of Medicine. Since the school was initially small, the chairman of the Department of Psychiatry was placed on all committees. The chairman planned the general medical orientation for the charter class of medical students. As a result, the students perceive psychiatrists as physicians keenly interested in teaching and in student activities. Being the only clinical department initially, major input from psychiatry was allowed in curriculum design, policy-making, search committees for all other clinical and some preclinical department chairmen, and class selection.

The College of Medicine utilizes community resources in its teaching program. Affiliation agreements to accomplish teaching goals have been established with three community hospitals: St. Joseph's Hospital, a private 600-bed acute care hospital; Tampa General Hospital, an excellent 800-bed municipal hospital; and the Veterans Administration Hospital, a 720-bed acute care hospital scheduled to open in the summer of 1972. The Department of Psychiatry opened in 1971 and is currently housed in a community mental health center located at St. Joseph's Hospital. This center has forty-four inpatient beds as well as the usual outpatient, partial hospitalization, emergency service, and consultation service components. Tampa General Hospital has a seventy-seven–bed psychiatric inpatient unit and a large outpatient unit. Two local guidance centers provide additional outpatient and children's services for the department's training programs. The new Veterans Administration Hospital has a 180-bed psychiatric inpatient unit and large day hospital and outpatient facilities. In addition, there are three thousand square feet of psychiatric research space and a large research budget. It appears that the intent of the Veterans Administration is to make this dean's committee hospital a national showcase of health care delivery.

In 1971, the American Medical Association approved a three-year residency training program in adult psychiatry and a two-year residency training program in child psychiatry. Two residents began training at that time. In July 1972, four new residents will begin the training program. In addition to the training of psychiatrists, the Department of Psychiatry is involved in supervising the multiinstitution, multiuniversity, and multijunior college affiliations needed for training mental health and allied professionals—medical students, psychologists, social workers, nurse clinical specialists, special education teachers, occupational therapists, rehabilitation counselors, gerontologists, pastoral counselors, mental health technicians, and the like.

The Department of Psychiatry was directed and staffed by one psychiatrist during its first year of existence. In the second year, an additional psychiatrist was added. In July 1972, there were nine full-time psychiatrists on the faculty. Within five years the department should include one hundred psychiatrists and numerous related mental health professionals. The staff is being selected on the basis of training and background, youth, enthusiasm, and the desire to be a participant in what promises to be a major innovative mental health program in this country. The basic orientation of the department is eclectic. Major emphasis will be on children, adolescents, and families. Excellent teaching will be the hallmark of the department.

Obviously, the crucial administrative problem to be solved is to make a workable, first-class training combination out of a large number of diverse clinical facilities. The newness of the College of Medicine and of the clinical facilities makes for a chaotic and often trying situation. On the other hand, it presents a tremendous opportunity to try some innovative ways of teaching, administrating, and providing clinical services.

Apart from the general guidelines set by the philosophy and objectives of the curriculum of the College of Medicine, the teaching philosophy of the Department of Psychiatry is generally based on current concepts of child, adolescent, and family psychiatry. There is a definite leaning toward brief, crisis-oriented and preventive-type intervention, whether for inpatients, outpatients, or partial hospitalization patients.

The medical school curriculum is generally aimed at providing clinical exposure as early as possible. It begins in the first week of medical school with the student simply mixing with the patients and conversing with them, thereby gaining a familiarity with the clinical problems. The first-year course gives instruction in interviewing and history-taking along with the didactic work in basic behavior sciences. This work includes such areas as human communication patterns, social group theory, marriage and family structure, sexual behavior, concepts of healing, ethnic and cultural differences, poverty, death and dying, and the meaning of hospitalization. Individual tutorial work is available for interested students and consists of an in-depth study of one patient and his family over a long term. As now proposed, the standard clinical clerkship will take place in the second- or the third-year course. The main points of emphasis will be: evaluation and management of psychiatric emergencies; practical psychopharmacology; and introduction to the process of psychotherapy, again emphasizing short-term intervention.

The residency curriculum is designed to begin where the medical student curriculum leaves off. In addition to emergency evaluation and management, supervised psychotherapy (short-term individual and family), and psychopharmacology, the resident is specifically instructed in the theory and practice of the inpatient milieu within the structure of a therapeutic community. The second year of residency is oriented to ambulatory care. The residents assume supervisory responsibilities for crisis-intervention workers and initiating conjoint therapy programs with other professionals. It is at this point that longer term individual and family therapy is taught and supervision provided. Instruction in group therapy and medical-surgical consultation are also begun this year. The third year of residency is elective. The resident may choose to spend a year of clinical administration, functioning as a ward chief supervising the day-to-day decisions concerned with patient care on his ward and supervising the first-year residents on that ward. Or he may elect to undertake a program of research, work toward a master of public health degree in community psychiatry, spend a year in child psychiatry, or explore other areas of interest. Didactic material is presented one day per week throughout the three-year curriculum and covers thirty-four areas of interest to residents, with the residents having significant input into the organization and modification of these courses.

University of Hawaii

Medical Student Teaching. We presently have a two-year curriculum school, and we are now actively planning for an M.D. degree-granting school for 1973. In the freshman year a first se-mester course in psychiatry focuses on the doctor-patient rela-tionship. A variety of contemporary medical-psychological-social problems are introduced in this framework, such as abortion (Hawaii being the first state to repeal its abortion law in 1969), organ trans-plant, and death and dying. Each student also has a tutorial ex-perience with a member of the clinical faculty, who interviews a patient with him. This specific in-depth doctor-patient relationship is then analyzed by the student in a paper turned in for evaluation. With the unique ethnic mix occurring among patients, faculty, and students in Hawaii the cross-cultural aspect of medicine in Hawaii is very important and is emphasized in our teaching in psychiatry. A psychiatrist actively participates in the medical course on history-taking and physical diagnosis. The sophomore year one-semester course on psychopathology continues emphasis on psychological medicine and clinical problem-solving. It exposes the students to the various psychiatric disorders by focusing on symptom syndromes of current sociopsychological medical importance, such as child abuse, delinquency, drug abuse, suicide, alcoholism, family problems, medical-surgical consultation problems, and emergency room practice. These too are considered in a cross-cultural, socioeconomic framework in order to highlight the need for flexibility of understanding and approaching patients and their families in medical practice. Each weekly two-hour session focuses on a clinical presentation worked up by the three or four students under the guidance of a faculty member who is an "expert" in that area. They review the literature and present a comprehensive overall view of the subject as well as relevant clinical material to highlight their presentation. The latter part of the session is devoted to class discussion. In working up the presentation, the students are actively involved in appropriate communtiy life experiences surrounding that particular topic, in order to understand their subject from an applied as well as a theoretical point of view and to communicate this to their classmates—they may visit a prison to learn about violent offenders, a "gay" bar and nightclub for sexual deviation, and so on. In our sophomore course, the stage is being set for the future junior clerkship (five weeks full time in psychiatry planned for 1973), which will utilize such settings as they are exposed to in the sophomore year, such as emergency rooms, family planning clinics, the child abuse center, neighborhood drug clinics. The department has also offered electives to the students in drug abuse, alcoholism, and cross-cultural psychiatry. Each year several students also elect psychiatry for their graduation thesis. Each summer an NIMH fellowship program in psychiatry is offered.

Residency Training. In 1969 the department, in its first year of full-time operation, assumed responsibility for the already existing residency training program in Hawaii. This program was reorganized as a three-way partnership of the oldest and largest nonprofit hospital in the state, the State Division of Mental Health, and the University of Hawaii School of Medicine. It now functions as the single accredited residency training program in the state, under the title "University of Hawaii Affiliated Hospitals." The program has approximately twenty residents in its three years of basic training assigned to all three basic training sites. Each of these sites offers a different clinical emphasis: inpatient, outpatient, emergency, and medical consultation services; community consultation experience with courts, correctional institutions, community drug clinics, and schools; and child and adolescent psychiatry. Residents are assigned an integrated and graduated sequence of these clinical experiences during their three years which provide supervised clinical contact with patients in a variety of treatment settings.

Child Psychiatry. A strong emphasis of the department is child psychiatry, particularly cross-cultural aspects of child development, psychopathology, and family functioning. The four child psychiatrists and the cultural anthropologist on the faculty reflect this emphasis. As in the basic program, the resident's patient population as well as his professional and nonprofessional colleagues comprise a balance of different ethnic groups and cultures: Caucasian, Japanese, Chinese, Portuguese, Filipino, Hawaiian, Samoan, and mixtures, as well as the blending by acculturation of serial generations of these groups. Much of his training focuses on differences in child-rearing, expression of illness, and therapeutic techniques adapted to cultural set and style of the family. The program, now in its first year of operation, has two third-year fellows in child psychiatry. It is planned that the program will provide the training arm and lead in the development of a consortium uniting the State Mental Health Association, the State Division of Mental Health, Kauikeolani Children's Hospital, and the University of Hawaii Department of Psychiatry, each of whose highest priority is the development of children's programs in Hawaii. The setting will be a comprehensive network of children's services developed through the work of this consortium. The first year comprises a basic orientation to child psychiatric practice. Readings are discussed with demonstration focusing on the psychiatric examination of children, diagnosis and classification, and treatment planning, followed by an intensive introduction to child development including preschool and newborn nursery observation, parenthood, and family functioning. This seminar shifts to weekly sequences in child psychopathology, child development, and the varieties of child therapies. Clinical experience parallels these sequences. The basic seminar in the second year of child fellowship will be in community child psychiatry, emphasizing the most recent developments in child mental health from population and systems approaches to community and consultative roles, and to prevention and child advocacy.

Throughout the two years a research and study emphasis on clinical experience will be based in community agencies. Cross-cultural aspects of child development and child psychopathology tie this program in with the department's first efforts in international psychiatry. An advanced seminar is aimed at extending understanding of family structure, child development, child-rearing and psychodynamics of children, normative and deviant behavior in psychopathology among children, and of the cross-cultural perspective. The seminar tries to teach child development and psychopathology by focusing on the range of differing behaviors as they emerge from culture rather than as parallel schools of thought. It examines familiar behavior in the Honolulu community among different ethnic groups, viewing its significance against a cross-cultural perspective, and also discusses normative behavior from country to country, particularly in the Pacific and Asia, and the need for assessing the development of child psychiatric services on the basis of existing knowledge of children in these countries. Several department members have helped to develop a demonstration training program for two psychiatrists from the University of Indonesia who have completed their three-year basic residency training in general psychiatry and who will train in child psychiatry in this program in 1972–1973. As a joint project between the University of Hawaii and the University of Indonesia, its immediate objective is to teach basic child psychiatry skills which can be applied regardless of social and cultural context and to focus on problem areas particularly relevant in that country, such as mental retardation and increasing delinquency. Its long-range objective is to research the nature and kinds of problems for which preventive and treatment programs need to be developed in Indonesia and to develop child psychiatry services in clinics and community settings in Indonesia. Although separate from the third-year fellowship in child psychiatry this program will be related to it and trainees will be paired as well as combined in the study-discussion group.

Southern Illinois University

Medical School Curriculum. The medical curriculum is founded on the principles of early and continuing clinical experience in a basic science orientation toward medical practice and real-world situations. Health maintenance and health care planning and delivery systems are important immediately. Emphasis is on learning and the concept of mastery rather than on being able to regurgitate a given percentage of the factual information presented in a classroom.

An organ-system approach will be used from the very beginning of medical school. Seventeen task forces have been appointed and are defining the educational objectives and content of the material that they propose to present in their particular organ system. Each task force is composed of basic scientists, clinical faculty, and practicing physicians. The various task forces are as follows: nervous system (including behavior and ethology), locomotor system, digestive system, excretory system (including acid-base balance and electrolytes), endocrine system (including reproduction), integumental system (including hair, nails), respiratory system (including medical ecology), circulatory system (including lymphatics), hematologic system, microbiology and immunology, cellular biology (including work on entry-level material that will be provided by other task forces), medical sociology (including medical economics), rudiments of history-taking, and physical examination and use of associated tools, emergency medicine and forensic medicine, health care planning (including general systems theory, Key Factor Analysis logic), collection and interpretation of biological data (including biostatistics, homeostasis, biologic rhythms), and the history of medicine. In addition to these specific curricular exposures, the student will have patient contact in a limited fashion from the very first week of medical school and continuing throughout the first year. He will also be taught the proper management of common emergency procedures. Specific time has been delegated to instruction in the health care delivery system. Medical sociology and psychiatry will also receive curriculum time, but wherever possible, these subjects will also be integrated into the organ-system approach. Interviewing techniques and patient contact will also be integrated into this approach.

The second-year curriculum will recapitulate the organ-system method of the first year. However, this time the approach is going to be disease-oriented and will occupy only about half of the second year. Second-year students will have a required ambulatory experience in family practice one afternoon a week for six months. This experience will take precedence over all other instruction. Thus, if the student is attending a conference or a lecture and one of his patients appears in the ambulatory setting, he will be called to attend that patient. Also during the second year there will be an intense undifferentiated clinical clerkship, during which the student will have an intensive, uninterrupted, six-week, full-time exposure to physical diagnosis. As currently envisioned this clerkship will be intense undifferentiated clinical clerkship, during which the student will have the opportunity to work-up one or more patients who demonstrate individually failure of one of the major organ systems. Thus each student will work-up a patient with liver failure, a patient with heart failure, a patient with chronic pulmonary disease, a patient with renal failure, and so on.

During the latter part of the second year, students will begin their clinical clerkship in the various disciplines. A student who has evidenced particular interest in one specialty will be allowed to take that clerkship first so that he may make a final decision that will guide him in selecting a residency. Obviously, all the major disciplines, including family practice, will be included in the clinical clerkship rotation.

Psychiatry. The chairman of the Department of Psychiatry arrived in August 1972. Psychiatry will be included in all phases of the curriculum in each of the three years, with a required six-week clerkship the third year. With respect to the family practice residency, psychiatry will have a major teaching responsibility, taking the form of ongoing supervision of the resident in his management of psychiatric cases one afternoon per week for each of the last two years of the three-year residency program. In addition, weekly seminars and lectures will be given on various topics of particular interest to the family physician. Time will be allocated to the behavioral sciences in the form of one hour per week for a period of six months during the residency.

Louisiana State University–Shreveport

The school's special orientation is centered around the concept of comprehensive care, for which a five-story building is being provided. Medical students will be assigned patients and families to follow continuously during their third and fourth years with collaborative available from all necessary services.

Medical students presently are given twenty-four hours of classroom time in each year. Thus far the curriculum has been fairly conventional, with lectures, clinical presentations, and some audio-visual material. The first year in psychiatry is devoted to "normal" psychological development and behavior and the second to psychodynamics and psychopathology. In the third year all students rotate through a six-week psychiatric clerkship on the inpatient psychiatric service at the Confederate Memorial Center. Students in the third year have one six-week block for an elective. The fourth year in psychiatry will include four weeks at the Mental Health Center working with a team on outpatient care. All students in the fourth year will have one four-week elective.

Residents spend the first year on the inpatient services of the affiliated hospitals. Second-year time is divided equally between inpatient work and outpatient work as a member of one of the treatment teams at the Mental Health Center. The third year is spent entirely at the Mental Health Center. During the third year the resident is assigned to neurology part time for two months and has two months in which he may do a full-time elective.

Michigan State University

The developing Health Sciences Center has several special characteristics. First, it is functionally integrated with the university. The joint administration of the basic science departments prevents proliferation and duplication of such departments. Joint appointments and joint administration has led to productive and effective relationships with all parts of the university.

Second, the role of the behavioral and social sciences is unusual. In 1964 the departments of anthropology, sociology, and psychology were incorporated into the administrative structure of the medical school in the same fashion as the traditional biological sciences. Members of the social science departments participate in all facets of committee work, including curriculum planning, teaching, and research in the college. In addition, many social and behavioral scientists have joint appointments within the clinical departments of the college and in its offices OHSER and OMERAD. A sociologist is associate dean of the school and works toward developing and maintaining social science contributions to programs of the College of Human Medicine.

The third special characteristic is depth of community involvement. From the beginning the teaching of behavioral and social sciences was carried out in the "community laboratory." Community hospital relationships, begun then, have since been developed as sites for clinical clerkships. Thus, beginning approximately twenty-one months prior to graduation, students move to clinical clerkship sites in Grand Rapids, Lansing, Flint, and Saginaw, where they complete their clinical training. Some full-time faculty are located "in situ" at these sites, supplemented by clinical (voluntary) faculty members and regularly scheduled visits from faculty members based on the campus. Psychiatry clerkships and liaison psychiatry programs have been or are being developed in each of these cities. Programs are jointly administered and funded by community educational corporations and the university.

Research in medical education is another special feature. The Office of Medical Education Research and Development (OMERAD) was founded in 1966. Its director, Hilliard Jason, was the first psychiatrist to come to Michigan State, though there was as yet no Department of Psychiatry. OMERAD has led the way in research on teaching and learning in medical schools, on the physician's diagnostic inquiry process, and in setting the tone for curricular planning, assessment of student progress, and the development of instructional objectives.

Research and education in health services are also emphasized. In July 1970 when funds became available for expansion to a four-year, degree-granting program, the medical school had Departments of Medicine, Psychiatry, and Human Development (Pediatrics). At that time, an Office of Health Services Education and Research (OHSER) was founded in addition to a Department of Surgery and a Department of Obstetrics, Gynecology and Reproductive Biology. OHSER has responsibility for studying and helping improve patient care and health services. Thus, the work in developing clinical facilities on campus and with community hospitals and agencies elsewhere will include evaluation and guidance from

OHSER. OHSER has also assumed responsibility for Regional Medical Programs. OHSER and the Department of Psychiatry are engaged in collaborative studies on the social and cultural epidemiology of heart attacks and coronary artery disease, as well as on the development of modular mental health manpower programs for the community. In addition, many members of the Department of Psychiatry are engaged in research bearing on the social, psychological, and cultural aspects of medical care systems, health and illness, and medical education.

Medical Student Education. Working closely with OMERAD, each department is developing instructional objectives for a three-phase curriculum that will not be tied to any specific length of time spent in medical education. Phase I will ordinarily be ten weeks in length and required of all students. Its implementation will be the responsibility of the Office of Interdepartmental Curriculum, a unit of the dean's office responsible for coordinating all interdepartmental and interdisciplinary educational programs. All departments contribute manpower to Phase I, which emphasizes the skills and knowledge necessary to interview patients, gather data, and undertake the problem-solving of clinical medicine. Phase I education is done in small groups with preceptors and includes a number of community experiences. An additional central purpose of this phase is the comprehensive evaluation of the student's capacities, areas of strength, and learning style, so that a program which is optimally adapted to his or her needs can be designed. Phase II is of indeterminate length. It corresponds to what is sometimes called "preclinical" education, although it involves a great deal of clinical exposure and experience, without students' taking individual responsibility for patients. The major element in Phase II is an educational sequence called Human Biology and Behavior, a multidisciplinary program involving all the basic and clinical departments. The objectives are designed by each department and coordinated by the curriculum committee. A variety of educational offerings are being keyed to these objectives, including self-instruction, small-group seminars, larger group meetings, and ready availability of academic advisors. In addition, many of the educational objectives are met in focal problem-solving exercises. These focal problems are built around a topic which may be a presenting problem to a physician.

The logic of solving the problem coupled with the knowledge needed to solve the problem make up the focus of these three-day, small-group learning experiences that are taught by interdepartmental groups of clinicians and basic scientists. The student will be able to proceed through Phase II at his own rate and present himself for assessment when he and his academic advisor agree that he is ready. Assessments are directly related to the educational objectives. A list of these objectives is furnished each student when he enters medical school. Once he has passed these assessments, he may proceed to Phase III, which is roughly comparable to clerkship in medical education. Phase III (like Phase II)` is completely elective. The objectives are furnished to the student. His program is then planned with his academic advisor. He may present himself for assessment when he feels he is ready. On passing the assessments, he will be granted the M.D. degree at the next commencement exercises. It is likely, once in full operation, that we will be graduating students at each of the four commencements each year. The Department of Psychiatry has developed most of its Phase III objectives and many of its Phase II objectives and is currently field-testing its assessment instruments.

Residency Training. In keeping with the medical school's principles of developing training programs in community agencies, our first residency program in collaboration with Pontiac State Hospital was initiated in 1969. The first residents under the new university-affiliated residency began in July 1970. Three residents are now in their second year and three in their first year. One division of Pontiac State Hospital, the North Oakland Community Mental Health Center, which is both state and federally funded, is the locus for the training in Pontiac. The residents spend one day a week at the East Lansing campus for seminars and supervision. AMA approval for a three-year residency program was granted in 1971 for training sites in Lansing and Flint. The Flint program will be carried out in the facilities of the Genesee County Community Mental Health Services, with inpatient services available in one or two community hospitals, or in Pontiac State Hospital, which is the Genesee County Services' regional hospital. Residents began training in July 1972 at Flint. The policy of the department has been one of gradual and careful growth consistent with our manpower and expertise. Therefore, active residency training in clinical settings in Lansing will probably not be initiated until 1973.

The University of Minnesota–Duluth

The objectives of the medical school at the University of Minnesota–Duluth can be summarized in four basic components: to increase the number of physicians trained in Minnesota; to emphasize a broadly based preparation for family practice (general practice/primary care) in the training program; to emphasize preparation for rural as opposed to urban practice; and to increase the likelihood that students trained in the Duluth school will remain in Minnesota to practice in communities with the greatest need.

In developing a primary/generalist curricular model for basic sciences teaching, two important concepts have evolved. First, basic science learning is critical to effective clinical medical practice and, second, the student's decision (and probably his actual ability) to remain a generalist is made early in his education. This decision must be reinforced by specific educational methods, procedures, and course content.

Clinical medicine consists of basic science and behavioral science applied to a patient and his problem. It is inevitable that basic science knowledge will change, hence that clinical practice will change. Students must adjust to this change continuously after graduation; they can do this effectively by being well-trained in current basic science. *De novo* learning or learning without a previous adequate base is neither efficient nor really possible. The Duluth program questions the progressing deemphasis of hard-science teaching in many curricula, considers this an overreaction, and is attempting to anticipate what the new equilibrium will be in 1980. Hopefully, we can reflect this future balance in our 1972 curriculum.

Career choices depend on many features of past experience, including certain self-perceptions and psychological introjects formalized well before primary school years. In order to retain a significant number of students in a generalist role the program must take these factors into account, provide adequate role preparation for students, and support them in the performance of that role once in practice. This supportive procedure will probably result in the student's being retained in the desired role rather than deviated into a new channel when he or she is well along in professional education.

Education for generalism in the Duluth program will consist of accurate identification of the basic scientific principles which constitute unifying factors in any group of scientific disciplines, together with the active teaching of these principles to students. Use of these principles in problem-solving is part of active teaching and is practiced until proficiency is achieved. An example is knowledge of the way antibiotic groups operate, whether by interfering with cell-wall synthesis, interfering with ribosmal protein synthesis, by competitive interference in cell metabolism, or by other mechanisms. Such knowledge permits intelligent selection of antibiotic pairs of new drugs once microbial resistance to a particular compound develops.

The nature of the teacher-student "contract" must be absolutely clear to both parties. Curriculum goals together with the nature of the role for which students are being prepared must be developed with students so that they understand them fully. The generalist role involves mastery of the central principles of each major medical discipline, competence in their application in problem-solving, and a specific level of detail knowledge to let the practitioner handle frequently occurring conditions without referral. Teaching detail knowledge in any discipline must stop at the level where definitive treatment of any patient would occupy an inordinate proportion of the physician's time, preventing his functioning as an effective primary physician for his other patients. These exclusions of care (such as management of an acute myocardial infarction, prolonged reoperative or postoperative care, control of the juvenile diabetic) must be clearly understood by the student, and the manner by which he can transfer patients to others for such care should be taught as one would teach any other care delivery principle.

Components of the curriculum are shown in Table 1.

University of Missouri–Kansas City

Educational Plan. The program for psychiatric training can best be presented by first describing in some detail the educational plan of the medical school. The overall objective, stated simply, is

Table 1

SCHEMATIC OUTLINE OF DULUTH CURRICULUM

FIRST YEAR—42 Weeks (Three and One-half Quarters)

Basic Science Component (7 weeks)	*Behavioral Component*	*Clinical Component*
Introductory period: Core morphology, chemistry, physiology, epidemiology	Physician's role Group processes Communication Interview	History and information Communication with patient

System Teaching (35 weeks)		
Neurobiology Cardiovascular Respiratory Gastrointestinal Renal Musculoskeletal Endocrine Reproductive	Mental function Cognition; intelligence Behavior as a learned phenomenon Emotions Motivation	Physical diagnosis and normal human state

SECOND YEAR—36 Weeks (Three Quarters)

Basic Science Component	*Behavioral Component*	*Clinical Component*
Introduction to pathology, microbiology and pharmacology (8 weeks)	Social aspects of disease	Introduction to clinical medicine
Infectious diseases (28 weeks)	Rural and urban social systems Social psychology Unusual development— retardation and the gifted Aging	
Abnormality in systems Nervous system Cardiovascular Respiratory Gastrointestinal Endocrine Genitourinary Blood and Lymph Skin Musculoskeletal	Abnormal behavior Social factors in mental health Introduction to clinical psychiatry	

to prepare students to become adequate physicians. In an effort to accomplish this goal, a six-year school has been created, thus permitting academically able students to enter directly after graduation from high school. (Students are admitted simultaneously to the medical school and to the undergraduate [arts and sciences] school of the university.) Further, an environment that resembles the practice of medicine as it exists outside the walls of the university is being designed. The establishment of the traditional departmental structure has been purposely avoided. In its place, several councils have been created: the council on Selection; the Council on Evaluation; the Council on Curriculum; and the Council on Docents. Faculty members from the medical school and the university are elected to these councils. Each council has a permanent member who holds the rank of assistant dean.

The function of the councils is implied in their respective titles. The Council on Selection selects faculty and students, the Council on Curriculum establishes curriculum, and the Council on Evaluation regularly evaluates student progress and curriculum quality. The Council of Docents consists of eight senior docents who review immediate teaching problems and concerns. A Coordinating Committee with members from each of the councils ensures cooperative functioning.

The councils are responsible to a dean, who is in turn responsible to the Office of the Provost of the School of Health Sciences (Medicine, Dentistry, Pharmacy, Nursing). Administrative support is provided the councils through an Office of Medical Education which is a part of the structure of the dean's office.

A core medical school curriculum has been established based on what a student is expected to learn within a six-year period. It is constantly updated and is known to the student body. The basic sciences, with a few exceptions, are not taught as separate entities but as part of the general medical school curriculum. First-year students spend thirty-six weeks in the undergraduate school of the university and the equivalent of twelve weeks in the medical school. This proportion is repeated in the second year. From the third through the sixth year, thirty-six weeks are spent in the medical school and twelve on the liberal arts campus. The curriculum in the first two years principally prepares the student for medical school, while in the remaining time a wide range of undergraduate and graduate courses is available. At the end of the six years a student can earn a baccalaureate degree as well as a medical degree.

Medical courses, all of which are taught to small groups of eight to ten students, from the outset involve patient presentations, history-taking, and physical exam demonstration and discussion, in order to illustrate the constant emphasis on clinical material. Both patient demonstrations and assignments provide direction in the study of specifically related segments of the basic sciences.

Beginning with the third year, students are assigned in groups of twelve to a team, lead by a docent, which is responsible for the full care of patients on its service for a twelve-week period. The term *docent* literally means teacher, in this instance a physician, clinician-scholar, usually an internist. The docent assumes primary responsibility for the education of the student for the remainder of his medical school career, and the student remains attached to his docent team even while assigned to other areas.

Psychiatric Instruction. The Curriculum Council believes that the teaching of psychiatry totally outside the context of other medical subject matter does a disservice both to medicine and to psychiatry. The introduction of psychiatric course material from the freshman through the senior year has not counteracted this tendency, since the traditional way to present this material is in blocks of time separate from other medical specialties or disciplines. This separation is of course also true of other specialty instruction. Thus, the student tends to compartmentalize, and the overall assimilation of the many facets of medicine into a meaningful gestalt, if it does occur, is achieved principally, and often painfully, through his own efforts.

It is also a well-documented fact that entering medical students demonstrate considerably more compassion and feeling for patients than do senior or graduating students. Teaching psychiatric principles that are useful in approaching and working with patients in general might well offset this tendency toward decreasing empathy.

The expectation at the end of six years is that the student will be familiar with and can utilize those basic psychiatric principles and techniques that allow him to deal comfortably, and at a defined level of competence, with a wide variety of patients. Further, he is expected to accept the presence of psychic and psychosocial factors, to a greater or lesser degree in all patients, as an inescapable fact of medical practice for whose management he possesses a degree of skill and acumen.

Psychiatry, then, participates in those teaching and service activities in which pertinent decisions are made about the diagnosis and care of patients. It also helps to construct the course content of the "formal" subject matter that is presented. There is consistent emphasis on helping the student recognize and understand those emotional and social factors that coexist with, are a result of, or contribute to the pathophysiological process under consideration.

In order to meet these aims, psychiatry is involved in the following ways. In the first year, a psychiatrist is assigned to each small group of entering students and participates no less than once weekly in the Introduction to Medicine as coinstructor. His involvement is generally during that period in which the historical material relating to the patient and his illness is discussed. The instruction is simple with a minimum of psychiatric jargon. Maximum student participation is encouraged, and students are helped to arrive at their own answers in regard to the understanding of pertinent or related emotional factors.

During the second year, the psychiatrist participates in both segments of Introduction to Medicine in the same way he does in the first year. Since presentations are more specialized here, psychiatric involvement is similarly defined. The emphasis remains on concept formation rather than principally on content. Instruction in medical interviewing and physical examination is provided by psychiatry and other specialties beginning in the third year!

In the third through sixth year a psychiatrist is assigned to each docent team and spends from eight to ten hours (over a two- to three-day period) in teaching rounds, with individual students or small groups of students. Since students have a variety of assignments following the twelve-week period with their docent team, a once-weekly seminar for each team with the team psychiatrist is being considered.

In the fifth year, thirty-six Saturday morning sessions of four hours each have been set aside for teaching behavioral science material. The Core Curriculum Manual will serve as the basis for the content of these sessions.

Mount Sinai

The Mount Sinai School of Medicine was established in 1963. The facilities of the Mount Sinai Hospital, which had been in existence for more than a century, form an integral part of the new medical school. During 1970–1971 the total enrollment was 164, with forty-one first-year students, forty second-year, forty-eight third-year, and thirty-five fourth-year students. The medical school is immediately contiguous to the hospital, which is located on the Upper East Side of Manhattan in an area which merges into East Harlem with a population primarily Puerto Rican and black. The hospital has a capacity of 1,300 beds, 103 of which are located on the Psychiatry Service. With the development of the medical school, a Basic Science Building was added to already existing facilities so that laboratory and classroom space for the basic sciences was available. The medical school has affiliations with the Beth Israel Hospital; Elmhurst Hospital in Queens, a city hospital; and a Veterans Hospital in the Bronx.

There are currently forty-five psychiatrists assigned to the Liaison Service and working in all other parts of the hospital, in addition to approximately 110 psychiatrists working within the Psychiatric Service. The existing beds are divided among four adult inpatient units and one child unit. The adult inpatient service admits patients from ages thirteen to ninety and includes a mixture of private and service patients on the same units. Thus, patients of various socioeconomic and ethnic backgrounds are available for teaching and service purposes. The inpatient child unit has fifteen beds and accepts patients from ages four to thirteen. An active psychiatric outpatient clinic gives attendings and residents opportunities to provide long-term psychotherapy, short-term psychotherapy, crisis intervention, aftercare, group psychotherapy, medication clinics, and the like, as well as maintains a twenty-four–hour emergency room service manned partly by attendings and residents. All these facilities are available for teaching psychiatry to medical students.

The curriculum of the School of Medicine provides for a

close integration of preclinical and clinical sciences. Emphasis is on the psychosocial aspects of disease and medical care and the application of modern medicine to the delivery of health care.

The framework of the curriculum in the first two years includes instruction in the basic sciences of anatomy, biochemistry, genetics, microbiology, pathology, pharmacology, and physiology. This is followed by integrated interdepartmental teaching of organ systems or clinical disciplines. The Department of Psychiatry, and specifically the Human Behavior Program, plays an active role in the integrated teaching. In addition to block time (department) and interdepartmental instruction in basic medical sciences, the programs of the first two years provide early exposure to clinical medicine and substantive periods of elective free time. The student may pursue various elective studies offered both by the School of Medicine and by the undergraduate and graduate institutions of the City University of New York.

The programs of the third and fourth years permit intensive study in direct patient contact, in seminars and demonstrations using the extensive facilities of the Mount Sinai Hospital and affiliated hospitals. Each student follows a complete rotation through various specialties and disciplines in the clinical services, including psychiatry and community medicine, during the third year and the first portion of the fourth year. This program enables the student to consider possible postgraduate career choices as he extends his knowledge and experience. The major portion of the fourth year provides elective time for concentration in a medical specialty or for research in the preclinical or clinical sciences.

The general objective of the undergraduate Human Behavior Program of the Department of Psychiatry is to familiarize the student with the nature, origins, mechanisms, and consequences of human behavior manifested in health and disease. A major training objective is the integration of biological, psychological, and social considerations into the general understanding and practice of the physician in relation to health and illness. Another important and critical objective is the presentation of the scientific basis of human behavior and the scientific methodologies employed. In view of these goals, the major teaching of human behavior is done on an integrated and interdepartmental basis.

In the first two years the psychiatric service is involved in teaching several interdisciplinary courses included in an integrated organ-system approach, in teaching various basic sciences such as pharmacology and physiology, in an Introduction to Medicine course, and in a Medical Ecology course. Thirty hours of behavioral science are taught in the second year under the direct auspices and supervision of the Department of Psychiatry.

In the third and fourth year, the medical student has clinical clerkships in the various departments of the Mount Sinai Hospital and affiliated hospitals. A four-week clerkship in psychiatry includes a strong emphasis on the biological, psychological, and sociocultural factors in the life cycle of man as they relate to psychiatric disorders. In addition, to provide integration of the study and understanding of human behavior with other disciplines, the members of the Liaison Psychiatry Service are involved in clerkships on the other services in which they demonstrate the application of these principles in all other specialties.

Medical students have a total of three hundred hours of elective and free time during the first and second year, and a number of electives in the Psychiatry Service are available to them according to the level of their training and experience. Summer electives also are available during the first and second year. The fourth year of the medical school curriculum is mostly an elective year, and the Department of Psychiatry provides electives in clinical studies or research in a clinical or basic science sector of psychiatry.

In the residency program, there are a total of thirty-six residents, seven in child and twenty-nine in adult psychiatry. The residency training program provides a year of inpatient service on units directed toward a therapeutic-milieu approach. The second year is an outpatient year, allowing for long-term psychotherapy, short-term psychotherapy, crisis intervention, diagnostic evaluation, group psychotherapy, aftercare, and psychopharmacology. The third year of the residency is an elective year, with programs being worked out individually in terms of the interests of the specific resident. All work done by residents, whether on an inpatient or outpatient basis, is closely supervised: approximately one supervisory hour per patient per resident on the inpatient service, a similar ratio for long- and short-term psychotherapy cases, and one hour of supervision per four hours of diagnostic evaluation and group psychotherapy. In addition, didactic courses in all years teach psychodynamics, psychopathology, phenomenology, principles of psychotherapy, history of psychiatry, and so on.

University of Nevada–Reno

Consistent with the interdisciplinary approach of the School of Medical Sciences, the Division of Behavioral Sciences is responsible for all teaching in psychiatry, as well as in the social and behavioral sciences. Currently staffed by only two full-time faculty members, the division draws heavily on the personnel and resources of existing campus departments, as well as community hospitals, agencies, and practitioners.

Undergraduate Medical Teaching. The division has input into the undergraduate medical curriculum in two ways: (1) regular weekly, four-hour blocks of time throughout the first two years, devoted specifically to teaching behavioral sciences, and (2) intermittent introduction of relevant contributions at appropriate points throughout the basic biomedical and clinical science curricula. In addition, in keeping with the philosophy of a "school without walls," students are introduced from the beginning to clinical roles and experiences which will help them to integrate relevant knowledge from the social and behavioral sciences into the rest of the curriculum.

One objective of the first-year program is to prepare students to relate to and communicate sensitively and comfortably with patients during the course on physical diagnosis given in the second semester, as well as to function effectively and independently during the clinical preceptorship required of all students between the first and second years.

After searching for a functional method for relating and integrating defined knowledge, skills, and attitudes in this area, the division decided that together with graduate students in psychology, social work, and nursing, all medical students would undergo specific orientation to and training for crisis intervention during the first

semester. While the particular emphasis of this approach is on training for work in the local Crisis Call Center, the basic behavioral
objective is to enable students to develop an early capacity to ap-
praise and respond to emotional and social crises.

A small-group approach is employed, with early focus on self
and other awareness and interaction. Later aspects of the training
develop specific interviewing and intervention techniques, including
appropriate use of therapeutic and community resources. The problem-solving orientation is further enhanced by specific discussion of
several common areas in which crisis intervention is particularly
necessary—drug use and abuse, alcoholism, suicide, death and dying,
sexuality, and family and marital conflict. Thus, the emphasis of
the first semester is primarily experiential in nature, with content
deemed to be of secondary importance.

As a transition to the more content- and clinically oriented
second semester, during the month of January students are provided
with a series of "selectives," each of which involves an investment
of approximately thirty hours of time in an in-depth exploration of
a particular problem or group experience. These include volunteer-
ing for the Crisis Call Center or participating in regular or marathon
encounter groups, various drug abuse programs, or self-designed
projects.

During the second semester of the freshman year, the continuing weekly four-hour sessions are conducted in a local hospital
setting and include content-oriented presentations and demonstrations, followed by small-group discussions or patient interviews
illustrating or elaborating the problem areas covered. Major subjects
include personality development and functioning, normal and
deviant behavior, stress and coping mechanisms, psychosocial factors
related to health and disease, and further introduction to psychotherapeutic and other methods of behavior change.

Although the second-year curriculum is still being developed,
it is currently planned to include further didactic instruction and
readings in psychopathology and psychotherapy together with supervision of short- and long-term individual or group therapy in local
agencies and hospitals. During this year, students will also be able
to participate in small group discussions with local psychiatrists, as

well as to accompany and participate in Rural Mental Health Clinics throughout the state.

Throughout both years, the division presents regular lectures, demonstrations, or discussions on relevant areas being covered in the basic subject blocks. Thus, work on the psychosocial aspects of cardiac disease and open heart surgery is reviewed during the cardio-vascular block, while the economic, ethical, and emotional aspects of kidney transplant and dialysis are included in the renal block.

In general, it is expected that students leaving after two years will be able to perform adequately in an inpatient or outpatient psychiatric clerkship and to proceed directly into a final clinical year if necessary (in case of a three-year curriculum).

Community Medicine and Health Care. In the absence of regular faculty in this area, the division has taken over responsibility for planning and implementing the curriculum in the areas of com-munity and preventive medicine, health care, and public policy and legislation with regard to health. Field experience and service in rural and urban health settings are being planned in conjunction with representatives from these areas and will include students from nursing and the allied health professions as well. Thus, the inter-disciplinary health team concept, introduced during the Crisis Call Training of the first semester, will be expanded in the community medicine block.

Undergraduate Health Sciences Teaching (Preprofessional). The relationship of the Division of Behavioral Sciences and the School of Medical Sciences to the overall university Health Sciences Program is unique. The coordination of all undergraduate and preprofessional instruction in the health sciences means additional teaching responsibilities for the division. Together with faculty members from other divisions of the school and from other schools and colleges of the university, members of the division are responsi-ble for planning and teaching in certain core curriculum courses for all undergraduate majors in premedicine, predentistry, pre-pharmacy, nursing, medical technology, physical therapy, and health education. Among those courses for which the division carries major teaching responsibilities are the following, required of all under-graduates in health sciences: Introduction to Community Health,

Interpersonal Skills, and Community Health and Human Development.

State University of New York at Stony Brook

A medical education must provide the intellectual tools and attitudes essential to the later pursuit in depth of a large number of specialties which will be entered upon much sooner than is now the case. We must realize that each of the basic sciences and the clinical specialties has a varying utility for any student, depending on his later role in medicine. Two essential tools are fundamental for any field of medical specialization: the "language" of the basic sciences and the "language" of the clinical sciences. And they must be taught as just that, languages to comprehend a given field in medicine.

The first two years in such a system can be considered as a unit, extending from cellular concepts to tissue and system levels of organization and proceeding from normal to abnormal and thence to clinical manifestations. They would merge as introduction to the clinical language—how to collect data from the patient by interview, physical examination, and laboratory and how to analyze such data, order it into probabilities by the diagnostic process, and arrive at prudent decisions as to action by value judgments.

This introduction to the two essential languages need not consume more than two years on the average. The student should then be ready to make a selection of one of a number of alternate pathways to the M.D. degree. With the help of a faculty advisory committee he can select a "major" field adapted to his interests, abilities, and personality. An "undifferentiated pathway" or track can be also reserved for those who wish to postpone choice of a field for a time. The student who selects a clinical speciality can devote the next four years, under university aegis, and emerge as a clinical specialist, taking six years to accomplish what now takes an average of eight years.

After a student chooses a specific path, he returns to intensified contact with the basic sciences but only those relevant to his clinical concerns. The most effective stimulus to learning the basic sciences for a clinician is the usually belated realization of their significance for his functioning as a specialist.

Several features are necessary in a new curriculum. One is

early introduction to the patient, not only in the first year but perhaps even in the later premedical years. Another is an experience in the social, ecological, and epidemiological dimensions of health and illness, which has become essential for anyone in medical school who thinks seriously about the social responsibilities of the physician. A new curriculum also needs to allow entry of students having more varied backgrounds than is now the case. This goal can be accomplished by a system which permits entry at several points in the curriculum, admits to advanced standing, and allows for make-up of science background for those who wish to enter with majors in social sciences or humanities.

The first two years of the curriculum of the School of Medicine are designed, then, to help the student achieve certain goals or skills: development of the basic science language; development of the clinical science language; understanding of the health delivery system; practical experience in clinical medicine; practical experience in community medicine; and problem-solving in matters affecting the health of the community.

Educational Assumptions. The following points are central to the educational program in the Department of Psychiatry: (1) All human behavior is understandable as the result of a complex interplay of biological, psychological, and sociological forces. (2) There is a body of knowledge about human behavior. The integration of this body of knowledge into the education of the physician is essential to medical competence. (3) Human behavior must be understood in the context in which it is found rather than simply in terms of its normality and abnormality. (4) It is not useful to create a mind-body dichotomy. (5) Effective medical treatment is most likely to be rendered when the physician is aware of his patient's pshchosocial circumstances—family, economic, ethnic, educational, attitudinal, and religious background. These factors influence etiology, course, management, and prognosis of dysfunction. (6) Dysfunction in one family member or social unit may result from or profoundly affect others in the unit for whom the physician may have responsibility, including preventative measures. (7) Effective medical treatment rests on the physician's skill in establishing and utilizing the doctor-patient relationship. (8) Emotional and behavioral disturbances frequently come first to the attention of the nonpsychiatrist physician and can best be recognized and treated by him. However, there are situations in which the patient's care may be enhanced by psychiatric consultation. The physician should learn when and how to use such consultation.

Instructional Goals. Goals are divided into attitudes, skills, and content. As physicians we hope that our graduates will display in their care of patients empathic concern, involvement, astute and complete observation, avoidance of value judgments of the patient, and a personal sense of professional competence in confronting the complexities of humanistic medicine. We assist the student physician in developing a personal point of view as a doctor that represents a synthesis of all viewpoints to which he has been exposed yet retains a sense of openness to new ideas and a feeling of responsibility for contributing to such new ideas.

Paramount to the acquisition of skills is the approach to comprehensive care which regards patients as persons. The clinical skills that we expect students to acquire are interviewing; diagnostic evaluation; planning and management; therapeutic use of the doctor-patient relationship; and use of physiologic therapeutic modalities. There are also what might be termed "personal skills," including the enhancement of the effective use of the self in the therapeutic relationship as well as in relationships with patients, other professional persons, and staff as individuals and in groups.

Interviewing is a core skill in all the disciplines concerned with comprehensive health care. When the student appears in medical school, he possesses to some degree all the capacities involved in the interviewing transaction. He has learned to listen, to observe, to elicit and understand information, and to impart it to others. He also has some experience in forming relationships and in taking some responsibility for other people. Our task is threefold: (1) to identify and define those situations in which a formal interview occurs—with an individual, a family, or other group; (2) to clarify the goals to be achieved by interviewing, such as medical history-taking, diagnostic evaluation, or psychological appraisal; (3) to provide the instructional environment which will help the student to organize and define as well as to reinforce those capacities described above which he brings to the task.

Diagnoses are simply convenient ways of summarizing observations about patients and comparing these observations with those of others. The diagnostic evaluation should ideally include four separate diagnoses: medical, personality, psychiatric, and social.

Skill in planning and management means the student's capacity to use the information obtained in the interview and the diagnostic evaluation in order to establish a plan of action which will be appropriate for the therapeutic intent. This plan must represent a synthesis of the student's understanding of biological, psychological, and sociocultural factors.

The student also is expected to make therapeutic use of the doctor-patient relationship. Psychotherapy is one of the goals of the interview; that is, behavioral change rather than information retrieval is sought. Determining the context in which psychotherapy should be taught and the kinds of models of psychotherapy which are most useful is a fundamental concern. The student should be directed to the type of crisis intervention which will help him deal effectively with anxiety reactions, marital and sexual conflict, suicide, the postpartum patient, the surgical patient, and the like. The program should also include techniques suitable for supportive care of the long-term patient. Another important subject is milieu organization and its implications for health and disease, such as psychological and therapeutic factors in the physician's offices, the hospital ward, the intensive care unit, and the community.

Several physiologic treatment modalities are available. Although many of these are clearly within the purview of the psychiatric specialist, every physician should be able to effectively use the most universally applicable modalities, primarily the psychopharmacological agents. The student should also be skillful in assessing and utilizing the psychological as well as the pharmacological effects of medication.

Content goals are based on a patient-oriented curriculum. The person identified as the patient brings to the medical transaction many levels of adequate and inadequate functioning. Teaching in the Department of Psychiatry must be directed toward the understanding and management of human behavior and the characteristic ways by which individuals master their problems.

A primary goal is to present areas of knowledge that help make human behavior understandable: (1) developmental processes, including their biological, sociological, and psychological aspects; (2) elements of interpersonal behavior systems, beginning with the mother-child transaction and generalizing to family transaction, peer relationships, and the individual's interaction with the larger society; (3) environmental factors including community, social class, religion, education, economic status, culture and ethnic background; (4) physical, physiological, and chemical factors influencing homeostasis; (5) human ecology—that is, the ongoing adaptation of a human population in its total environment.

Interaction of the determinants of behavior is viewed relativistically so that the student avoids thinking in terms of absolute norms. A longitudinal vew is taken of the origin, course, and outcome of the patient's dysfunction. The student should be able to integrate and understand personal, family, and community resources leading to a rational program of treatment. He will develop awareness of his personal reaction to the therapeutic relationship and learn techniques in which the self is a therapeutic agent.

Other content areas to be covered are the theory and technique of interviewing and the conventional diagnostic categories. Diagnosis is considered incomplete unless it includes social, personality, medical, and psychiatric diagnostic features. Various psychotherapeutic models are presented to help the student find his own most effective methods of psychotherapy. Drugs and other physiological interventions are also emphasized. Finally, the student participates with and refers to other health professionals.

Medical College of Ohio–Toledo

The Department of Psychiatry is involved in curriculum planning and medical student education in all three years of the medical school education. In addition, independent and investigative study is chosen by many students with members of the department.

During the first phase, information on growth and development, cognitive development, social and psychological factors involved in illness and health, the doctor-patient relationship, and interviewing and history-taking are given in an interdepartmental fashion with major input from the Department of Psychiatry. We do not have a division of behavioral science but most of the material from this area is presented in this phase. In Phase II the chief departmental teaching is in two forms. One is a two-week block of time during the Nervous System and Behavior Sub-Committee which introduces psychopathology, diagnosis, and treatment modalities. This "miniclerkship" demonstrates interviewing techniques as well as some of the variations from normal to abnormal. The second form is through integrated teaching in other organ systems. For example, in the reproductive system a block of time is spent on human sexuality, including the biological, social, and psychological factors contributing to human sexual identity and behavior. During the renal system, time is spent on enuresis and on the psychosocial aspects of hemodialysis.

The department has a four-week mandatory clerkship during Phase III (we hope to get two more weeks). During this time the student receives experience with children, families, traditional psychiatric inpatients, and consultation patients (including suicidal, delirious, geriatric, psychosomatic, and management-problem patients). He learns some of the techniques and therapy as well as the diagnosis and consultation process. Additional emphasis is placed on history-taking, interviewing, and knowledge of community facilities. Some students elect additional time in psychiatry, which can be experience with outpatients, consultation, children, or adolescents or experience at St. Vincent Hospital.

Pennsylvania State University

The Department of Psychiatry is the last major clinical department to be established in the College of Medicine and Medical Center. Since its inception in July 1971, there has been rapid progress in faculty recruitment, development of a teaching curriculum for medical and graduate students, providing a full range of clinical services for psychiatric care, and development and continuation of highly sophisticated programs of psychiatric research.

The faculty of the Department of Psychiatry plays an important role in teaching the medical student, not only in the clinical years but also in the first two years. Required courses are taught by the faculty in three of the six quarters in the first two years. This teaching is integrated with that of the departments of Humanities, Behavioral Science, Family and Community Medicine, and Medicine. In the first year, students are taught various aspects of growth and development and interviewing techniques and are introduced to descriptive psychopathology and community psychiatry. The psychiatry curriculum in the second year includes the evaluation and treatment of psychiatric disorders, child psychiatry, community psychiatry, and psycho-biological-social research studies. In the third year, the student has four required weeks of psychiatry. Emphasis is on the student's evaluating and treating psychiatric patients under close supervision in a variety of settings. Formal teaching and clinical experience in community psychiatry are emphasized throughout the medical student's education. The Department of Psychiatry has also established a number of elective courses including: clinical electives in psychosomatic consultation, inpatient psychiatry, community psychiatry, and drug addiction; research electives related to the Sleep Research and Treatment Facility, the Neuroendocrinologic and Biochemical Correlates Laboratory, and the Performance Evaluation Laboratory; and a clinical research seminar on selected topics.

Graduate students from any of the basic science departments may elect to take any of the courses described under Medical Student Education. More important, a number of graduate students are actively involved in the Department of Psychiatry research programs in relation to work on their doctoral dissertations.

The overall objective of the Psychiatric Residency Program is to train physicians in all aspects of the general practice of psychiatry. This goal includes the understanding and treatment of mental illness, not only as it pertains to the individual but also to the community. In addition, residents obtain experience in academic teaching and investigative research. The interpersonal accessibility of all staff members is a major factor in the resident's gaining intensive support and supervision in his work with parents. The flexibility of the residency program offers opportunities and support for developing areas of specialization and for research interests. All department programs are interdisciplinary and all the mental health teams are trained in the same settings, in the same manner.

The three-year Psychiatric Residency Training Program is a balance between formal didactic course material and clinical experience. Training in community psychiatry occurs throughout the program. Residents also have opportunities to follow patients over the three-year period so as to gain a better understanding of the longitudinal aspects of psychiatric illness. A team approach is utilized in evaluating and treating patients; the team consists of a resident, staff psychiatrist, psychologist, psychiatric social worker, and psychiatric nurse. The primary purpose of the resident's clinical experience is training, not service. Residents obtain considerable staff supervision both individually and in small groups of two or three residents.

The first year emphasizes evaluation and treatment of inpatients on the adult psychiatry unit. Individual and family psychodynamics are stressed. In addition to the individual psychotherapies, there is considerable importance placed on group psychotherapy, milieu therapy, and treatment with psychopharmacological agents. Experience in community psychiatry includes learning about the various community resources and the follow-up and aftercare of discharged patients.

The academic curriculum in the first year is comprehensive and includes the following areas: personality development, introduction to psychopathology, psychotherapeutic techniques including psychodynamic approaches and behavior modification, psychological testing, somatic therapies, neurochemistry, psychopharmacology, social and community psychiatry, and psychiatric research.

In the second and third years, about half the resident's time is spent in supervised therapy of outpatients, both in the hospital outpatient clinic and in community mental health clinics. This includes supervised experience and training in family therapy and group psychotherapy. In the second year, the other half of his time is devoted to child psychiatry, community psychiatry, and neurology. In the third year in addition to the aforementioned outpatient work, half his time is occupied by electives and psychiatric consultation within the general hospital.

The department plans to have four residents in each of the three years. Four residents in the first year and three residents in the second and third years were accepted for residency training starting in July 1972. Current plans are for the child psychiatry residency training program to begin in July 1973.

General Consultation and Education. As previously mentioned, the training of all mental health personnel is integrated within the department and is interdisciplinary in nature. In the near future, training programs will be initiated in the department for social work, psychology, and nursing students. Emphasis will be placed on training graduate rather than undergraduate students in these fields.

Several community programs have already been established to provide consultation and education for mental health workers as well as police, teachers, probation officers, and others. As the efforts of the Department of Psychiatry and Harrisburg Community Mental Health and Mental Retardation Center become integrated the consultation and education programs will be further expanded. Currently, the department supports a monthly Distinguished Speaker's Series which may be attended by anyone with a professional interest in mental health. Conferences are also held for the purposes of inservice training of police and clergy. A three-day symposium, planned and supported by the department, assessed and evaluated overall community resources especially in the mental health area that exist in central Pennsylvania.

Rush–Presbyterian St. Luke's Medical Center

Undergraduate Program. The core courses for medical students are presented by interdepartmental "task forces" consisting of members drawn from the various departments of the college. From time of entry the student is intended to receive an interlocking program in scientific methodologies and experimental approaches and an introduction to patients and their problems. Opportunities and facilities for research in the biological and behavioral sciences, in clinical sciences, and in environmental biology are available in the various departments of the college.

The program importantly depends upon the interaction of a student and his principal advisor, whose primary responsibility is to help the student define his goals, become a person capable of independent and continuing study, and choose courses of study. The initial task of each principal advisor and his student is to identify past achievements, the strengths and weaknesses of the student. This evaluation process continues through the educational program pursued by each student. The principal advisor program is coordinated by the Office of Student and Faculty Affairs.

The educational program of Rush belongs to a continuum that emerges from an arts, sciences, and humanities experience and continues into years of practice, study, teaching, and inquiry. The program has three phases.

Phase I has three objectives. First, courses will provide the fundamental concepts and vocabulary on which the clinical sciences are based. Second, the student will gain understanding of the delivery of medical care, the interactions of society influencing health, and the study of man's behavior and his ability to communicate. Third, the student will begin to develop professional concepts and clinical skills under the continuing tutelage of an individual clinical tutor. This professional relationship endures through Phase I and Phase II, during which the attributes, attitudes, and abilities of a physician will be developed by the student. The content of the courses in Phase I is prerequisite to undertaking Phase II of the Rush program.

Phase II integrates basic and clinical sciences to provide an understanding of man in health and disease through a series of courses concerning the organ systems of the body. The quarters of Phase II do not imply a necessary curricular sequence, and one or more quarters may be omitted and the material covered in independent study. The theme of Phase II courses is to provide the basic information necessary to the functioning of all physicians, in a context relevant to the experience of each student with his clinical tutor; continual encounters with human disorders facilitate the student's acquisition of independent study techniques as he searches for answers to clinical questions.

Phase II is divided into four instructional units, each of which occupies an academic quarter. The winter quarter contains the task force courses on reproduction and maturation, including reproduction, growth development and behavior, and a course on the endocrine and metabolic systems. Spring quarter courses present the skin and neurosensory-communicative systems. The summer quarter contains courses pertaining to the locomotor, gastrointestinal and hemapoietic systems. Courses which deal with the excretory, respiratory and cardiovascular systems are included in the fall quarter of Phase II.

Phase III contains core clinical clerkships and elective periods. The initial experience in this phase for most students, the core clerkship is intended to develop the student's capability to elicit data from all sources pertaining to patients, to make meaningful diagnostic hypotheses, and to carry out necessary tests of hypotheses. During this experience the practice of scientific medicine is to be developed. The subsequent program recommended for most students will consist of core clerkships in medicine, surgery, pediatrics, psychiatry, and obstetrics-gynecology. Tentative or firm career choices modify the duration and types of clerkships and elective experiences of Phase III. Electives are designed to supplement the core portion of the educational program. The student and his principal advisor will devise an individual curriculum best adapted to his career goals. Unique educational experiences not listed in this portion of the educational program may be generated upon request of the student and his advisor. Details concerning the duration and times of availability of each course will be arranged with the individual course coordinators.

The flexible program of Rush Medical College permits a wide variety of career choices compatible with the broad spectrum of educational experiences pursued prior to matriculation at Rush.

Objectives of Psychiatry Courses. The Department of Psychiatry will teach the students how the biological, psychological, social, and cultural systems interact in the developing personality and its expression in behavior. We will help the student to systematically develop his identity as a physician, increase his powers of observation, and gather pertinent data. Students will be taught the following: a general systems frame of reference which will lead them to view disease as a multifactoral process; how the many systems interact in the disease process although specific systems may be predominantly involved; the significance of psychosocial and organic factors and how they interact in behavior disorders; the therapeutic significance of the doctor-patient relationship, the patients' social and cultural system, and the medical milieu on the hospitalized patient; and how to evaluate and manage behavior disorders.

Required Courses. In Phase I psychiatry faculty combine with faculty from other departments to teach a course titled Observation and Communication. Our objectives in this course are to develop the student's ability to establish rapport with patients and develop his powers of observation and pertinent data-gathering. These skills can then be utilized while interviewing and examining patients.

In Phase II an interdisciplinary course called Growth Development and Behavior is given by faculty from psychiatry and from several other departments. The objective of this course, totaling 128 hours, is to help the student understand how the various systems—biological, psychological, social, and cultural—interact as the developing human being proceeds through the various phases of his life cycle. The cyclical nature of the life cycle is emphasized. Also in Phase II several members of the department are teaching within the courses on the organ systems, including the reproductive, cardiovascular, gastrointestinal, and excretory systems.

In Phase III the department presents its basic clinical clerkship in psychiatry. Its aims are to provide the student with opportunities to better understand interpersonal relationships, to clarify and identify psychological phenomena as demonstrated in a number of psychopathologic states, to develop some competence in recognizing those conditions requiring more expert care, and to acquire confidence and ability to provide therapeutic assistance to those patients having accessible emotional problems. Direct experience with patients is provided wherever possible. The patient is seen, evaluated, and cared for as an individual living within a dynamic physical-social-cultural system wherein the various stresses are met through various psychological coping mechanisms. A preceptorship, an association with a staff member, takes place one whole day a week.

The student is given experience in all elements of the system of care: the community health center, the outpatient clinics for children and adults, the Day Hospital for Children, the Inpatient Services for Children and Adults, and selected other resources in the community. Electives are available in adult, child, community, and psychosomatic psychiatry and in psychotherapy.

Graduate Psychiatry. The residency training program is a broadly conceived and carefully executed program of dynamically oriented specialty training approved for three years as required for certification in psychiatry by the American Board of Psychiatry and Neurology. The number of residents is limited to four per year. An unlimited variety of clinical case material and the presence of a large teaching staff allow the program to be well-supervised and tailored wherever necessary to the needs of the individual resident.

The fundamental objective of the psychiatry residency program is the development of a keen spirit of inquiry into all aspects of human nature and behavior. Considerable emphasis is placed on understanding the interrelatedness of the individual, his group, his environment, and the community which surrounds him. The ultimate goal for the student is a psychodynamic understanding of behavioral and other phenomena which will then permit a high level of therapeutic skill. Basic knowledge is progressively enlarged upon by means of seminars, bedside teaching, clinic presentation, case supervision, and group participation. In this way each resident can define for himself the limits of what is known in the various areas of psychiatry and may begin to explore unknown areas of research interest.

The three-year program is a balanced one, with appropriate emphasis on diagnosis and treatment of inpatients and outpatients, both adults and children, lectures and seminars on somatic and psychological treatment, and individual and group supervision. The basic orientation of the department is psychoanalytic; however, a variety of viewpoints is represented among the staff so that training is comprehensive. There are other areas of experience to which each resident is exposed in addition to clinical and didactic training. The role of psychiatry in the community is stressed, taught by participating in or visits to facilities within the community or in community life. Opportunity is given each resident to develop consultative and administrative skills. Furthermore, residents are required to participate in the teaching program conducted by the department for nurses and medical students. The training scene includes a sixty-two–bed inpatient service, a developing mental health center providing all varieties of ambulatory care, and collaborating community facilities and institutions.

Child Psychiatry Training Program. The Section of Child Psychiatry offers a fully approved two-year residency in the subspecialty of child psychiatry. Two qualified candidates are matriculated each year. The program gives specialized training in the appropriate clinical, consultative, and administrative skills. The development of diagnostic and therapeutic skills, however, is but part of the total objective of this training program; a constant review of established ideas by staff and trainees is encouraged as an ongoing examination of the traditional theoretical models operant in the realm of child and adolescent development.

The inpatient and outpatient facilities for children are carefully integrated so as to provide a totally supervised program in which the resident is able to follow cases through all phases of patient care. In the outpatient service the resident works both independently and collaboratively with the staff in a multidisciplinary setting. By means of individual supervision and seminars he is introduced to the diagnostic and therapeutic processes involved in all aspects of screening and admission, the diagnostic evaluation, and the choice of therapeutic techniques. He works with the allied disciplines of psychiatric social service, psychology, pediatrics and neurology. Therapy cases are assigned so as to provide a variety of experience for each trainee, ensuring the development of a broad competence in all clinical areas. Supervision of treatment cases is provided generally with a ratio of one hour of supervision for three hours of therapy. Rotation through a Children's Day Hospital provides a close view of children having major behavior problems at home and in school.

The carefully organized Inpatient Service for Children and Adolescents allows for supervised training in intensive diagnostic and psychotherapeutic procedures, hospital management, and patient disposition. Opportunities for observation, investigation, and management of group relationships are provided.

During the second year of training there is a gradual shift of emphasis in both diagnostic and therapeutic work. In the outpatient clinic the number of diagnostic cases decreases, and the resident, with supervision, assumes responsibility for all phases of the evaluative procedure in each case assigned to him. He is given training, liaison, and consultative responsibilities. With supervision, he teaches medical students, interns, and residents from other departments of the hospital. Special emphasis is placed on consultation in both pediatric outpatient and inpatient services. Throughout his training the resident is taught the use of various treatment modalities including individual, group, and family therapy.

Experience is provided with special schools for the emotionally disturbed, the mentally retarded, and the multihandicapped child, placement agencies, day care centers, youth centers, residential homes for children, and the juvenile courts. During the second year of training opportunities are available for supervised consultative work in one or more of these agencies.

University of Texas–Houston

Organization. The educational program encompasses a period of three calendar years and consists of twelve instructional quarters of eleven weeks each. Approximately two months of vacation time are provided each calendar year. The first six quarters prepare the student for the specific clerkship experiences that comprise the seventh, eighth, and ninth quarters. During the first six quarters the student becomes familiar with the basic and applied biomedical sciences through lectures, seminars, demonstrations, tutorial sessions, and self-instructional aids. These learning experiences are presented as core interdisciplinary courses by appropriate members of the faculty working as teaching teams. As the student progresses from a study of the morphology of the human body and the fundamentals of molecular and cellular biology to that of the normal and abnormal structure and function of the various organ systems, he is introduced to the techniques of interviewing, history-taking, and performance of physical and mental status examinations. Similarly, he is given the opportunity to become proficient in working with the more common laboratory procedures and manipulating the resultant data. Appropriate materials from the behavioral and social sciences are presented concomitantly. During this portion of the curriculum, approximately three half-days a week are devoted to laboratory projects in which each student works in conjunction with faculty members in their laboratories. This type of laboratory experience supplements the more traditional standardized laboratory exercise approach.

After completing this educational sequence, which makes up the first half of the curriculum, the student is prepared to progress through a classic series of clinical clerkships for the next three quarters. These will include assignments to medicine, obstetrics and gynecology, pediatrics, psychiatry, surgery, and others.

The remaining three quarters in the curriculum present several track options, which include family practice, specialty practice, social and community medicine, behavioral science, and medical research. In consultation with faculty advisors each student devises an educational sequence that relates specifically to his ultimate career goals and to his postgraduate educational plans. Participation in one of these track options enables the student to demonstrate his acquisition of some expertise in one area of practice or scientific activity as a requirement for receiving the M.D. degree.

Psychiatry faculty are responsible for teaching behavioral science, psychology, social sciences, and psychiatry. The present curriculum includes forty hours of instruction in behavioral and social sciences during the third and fourth quarters. An additional thirty hours in the sixth quarter will be devoted to basic clinical psychopathology. During the core clinical curriculum psychiatry will have five weeks of the thirty weeks available. Students will devote three weeks to general psychiatry, one week to alcoholism, and one week to the problem of drug abuse. During the track option period there will be a behavioral sciences track in which the student can elect to spend thirty weeks in psychiatry. The program has not yet been formulated. In addition, psychiatry will have major input into the social and community medicine and family practice tracks. The major emphasis of the program in psychiatry will be biological with strong emphasis on social and community programs.

Residency Program. The university will shortly be submitting for approval a combined residency program for the major affiliated hospitals.

Texas–University of San Antonio

All course work is given in the first two years. The third year is entirely for clinical clerkships—fourteen weeks each on medicine and surgery and seven weeks each on obstetrics and gynecology, pediatrics, and psychiatry. The fourth year is entirely elective. Students may take on- or off-campus electives in clinical or basic sciences. A newly developed optional three-year curriculum began July 1972.

The Department of Psychiatry participates in the teaching program in all four years of the medical curriculum, primarily in courses given by the department, but also in task force teaching. In the first year, the department has responsibility for an eighty-four–hour human ecology course. During the first term of the course, students are assigned in groups of five or six to eighteen to twenty agencies within the community. At each agency, students are assigned four families with whom they work. The principal goal for the students is to gain firsthand observation of different life styles and situations. Students are required to make observations in the "natural" environment of families, to organize their observations, and to write them up in medically relevant terms. The majority of students respond positively to the experience. The second term of the course is conducted in the classroom. Theoretical and conceptual materials on human ecology are woven in among case materials and other presentations of social, emotional, and behavioral aspects of patient care.

The sophomore course in psychiatry, a sixty-nine–hour course given in the first four and half months of the academic year, is an introduction to descriptive and dynamic psychopathology and the role of psychological factors in the care of nonpsychiatric patients. The major objectives are to familiarize students with basic psychiatric concepts, methods, and information so that they are prepared for more intensive clinical studies in psychiatric and nonpsychiatric areas in the third and fourth years. This course includes training in interviewing techniques, dynamic understanding of the relation of earlier life events to current variables in psychopathogenesis, diagnostic characteristics of each psychiatric disorder, principles of therapy, the relation between psychological factors and somatic disease, and principles of managing situations in medical practice. Sixteen hours are devoted to small-group clinical teaching, in which live patients are interviewed by faculty and students. The remainder of the course involves the entire student group in the classroom. Didactic lectures, class discussion, handouts, text assignments, and the presentation of clinical material via television recordings, live patients, and movies are utilized.

The seven-week Junior Clerkship in Psychiatry includes clinical periods on the inpatient, outpatient, and child psychiatry services, as well as seminars and case presentations, covering a variety of psychiatric states, community programs, and theoretical concepts. Because of the size of the class, the clerkship has been divided into three sections, one of which has approximately 90 percent of its experience within an outpatient setting, including day hospital and screening programs in a mental health unit. The other two sections are trained in both the inpatient and outpatient services. Students in the outpatient section receive some inpatient experience on night call and weekend call.

With the establishment of TV equipment within the department, sections of the clerkship are devoted to recording students' interviews of patients on tapes which are played back to the students, allowing them to observe and improve their interviewing techniques.

Elective courses in both clinical and basic areas relating to psychiatry are offered. An attempt is made to work with the student and develop an elective in the area of the student's interest.

Residency Training. The Psychiatry Residency Training Program began in July 1969 with six first-year residents. We now have a total of fifteen residents in the first, second, and third years. The first group of residents completed their training in June 1972. A fellowship program in child psychiatry was developed in cooperation with the medical school, the Bexar County Teaching Hospital, the Community Guidance Center, and the San Antonio Children's Center. The latter offers residential and day care for emotionally disturbed children. There are now two child fellows in this program.

Residents begin training on a thirty-six–bed inpatient service which is oriented to short-term treatment and crisis intervention. For two half-days each week, residents rotate through several community programs such as alcoholism, drug addiction, and mental health field work in model cities areas. They also begin outpatient work with discharged inpatients. Because of a geographic separation of inpatient and ambulatory care, we have not been able to institute complete continuity of care.

The second year is spent in outpatient work, day hospital care, child psychiatry, and consultation service. In the third year, the resident has six months in a chief resident position on one of the services he selects. The other six months are elective.

Graduate and Postgraduate Education. We are in the second year of a training program in clinical psychology. In each of these years, we have had seven psychology residents in training for one year. These are psychologists who have either completed their Ph.D.s or completed the program for their Ph.D.s.

We also have a program for training medical sociologists. This is a joint effort of the Department of Sociology of the University of Texas at Austin and the Division of Sociology of the Department of Psychiatry in the medical school. Sociologists take graduate course work in Austin and then come to the medical school for a field experience and possibly to do their dissertation. There are now four students enrolled in the program. One of them is working at the medical school and the other three are in Austin.

Texas Tech University

General Medical School Program. The Department of Psychiatry is strongly oriented toward education of family physicians and toward community medicine. Innovative techniques of teaching will be used to help the student pursue areas of special interest and competence without sacrificing an average expectable competency in general psychiatry. A small-group, individually-tailored approach will be used throughout the program of instruction.

The psychiatric curriculum is predicated on a four-phase, thirty-six–month medical school experience. The thirty-six months run consecutively and are divided into fall, spring, and summer trimesters of four months each. Students complete four equal phases during three calendar years of study.

The fall trimester of the first year will provide the setting for the basic science of psychiatry. Basic behavioral science, personality theory, psychopathology, and history of psychiatry will be covered in this time period. The teaching of this material will require approximately one hundred hours. The teaching team will consist of psychiatrists, anatomists, physiologists, psychologists, sociologists, and anthropologists. Instruction will be carried out in seminars and small discussion groups. This block of instruction will equip the student with the basic tools necessary to progress to more integrated and more clinically oriented phases of his learning experience.

The second and third trimesters of the first calendar year should require no discrete psychiatric course per se. Department faculty will contribute to the clinical blocks of these trimesters by providing input that is integrated with basic sciences as well as other clinical sciences. The psychiatrist will be a member of the teaching team. This approach has the advantage of introducing techniques of interview, doctor-patient relationships, and psychosomatic concepts in a natural, appealing way to the student and reinforces the integrated team concept. This part of the psychiatric curriculum will be supplemented by reading lists and various other teaching aids (tapes, films, and so on) to be used at the students' discretion. The entire first year will be punctuated by examinations covering logical segments of information that have just been presented. In other words, when a segment such as psychoanalytic theory has been covered, an exam will be given. Challenge exams will be constructed for those students who feel competent in any segment of psychiatry to allow them to progress at their own rate of speed.

The second year of the medical school curriculum is divided into five major clinical modules—medicine, surgery, psychiatry, pediatrics, and obstetrics-gynecology—of eight or nine weeks each. One module provides the major psychiatric experience for the medical student. During this period, the student participates in small-group learning experiences embracing the entire field of clinical psychiatry. He is introduced to the psychiatric syndromes and becomes familiar with various forms of psychiatric treatment. He spends large segments of his time with psychiatric patients in hospitals and clinics. Psychiatry as it relates to family and community problems is heavily stressed. He also is allotted realistic amounts of time to pursue special interests within the field, under the guidance and supervision of a faculty member assigned to his small group for the duration of his group's psychiatric rotation.

The student will also spend time dealing with psychiatric emergencies (emergency room) and doing consultation within the general hospital. Community psychiatry will be introduced. By the end of his second year, he will have had a comprehensive, practical course in psychiatry, especially as it relates to medical practice in general, and should be able to decide whether he wishes to continue his study in this field by choosing a third-year elective.

The third and final year will offer several electives in psychiatry. Each should be a complete module, lasting from six to ten weeks. An elective in psychiatry should cover areas not previously dealt with in depth as well as intensify and lengthen the student's exposure to the general field of clinical psychiatry. The elective will be worked out by the student, the faculty member of his tutorial team, and an individual mentor from the department of psychiatry. Various research interests, child psychiatry, community psychiatry, and psychosomatic medicine are some of the areas that may be offered as "core areas" in an elective the third year. The core areas of study and experience will be supplemented by additional experience in clinic and hospital. The student is expected to write a paper dealing with his area of interest. This paper would hopefully be suitable for publication and would serve as an evaluation in lieu of examination.

The freshman classes of 1972, 1973, and 1974 will follow the psychiatric curriculum as outlined above. The first three "third-year" classes, which will be accepted in those years, present a problem in that they will come from various schools with different curricula. It is assumed all will have had some psychiatry. This assumption should be reinforced by a "crash" course in basic psychiatry consisting of five or six lectures followed by an assessment examination. Those students who are deficient in basic psychiatry will be dealt with individually in a remedial course (small-group tutoring) and, at the same time, will proceed with their classmates into the third-year course as outlined above. The same elective prerogatives will apply to these students in their fourth year that will obtain for our entering freshmen in their third and final year.

Curriculum Details. The following methods will be used to teach the basic didactic course in psychiatry (one-hundred hours): lectures, small-group discussions, seminars, movies, and televised patient interviews. The material covered during the first trimester will include (1) emotional factors in medical practice: biological, sociological, and psychological factors; (2) adaptation to stress, including techniques to increase adaptational abilities; (3) personality development; (4) psychodynamics of normal behavior, including psychoanalytic theory and adaptational dynamics.

The system for implementing the integrated team teaching approach will use an interlocking network of educational consultants. The chairman of psychiatry will either function as the educational consultant from psychiatry or will appoint one of his faculty. This man will consult with other educational consultants or representatives of other departments to coordinate teaching efforts. For instance, prior to the beginning of the academic year he will meet with the representative from the medicine department to coordinate areas in which psychiatry and medicine will interface. An example might be during a block when the department of medicine is covering coronary artery disease; psychiatric input would be valuable to the team teaching of this subject along with contributions from the departments of physiology and biochemistry. The various areas of interfacing should be worked out before the beginning of each academic year by the educational consultants or other representatives from various departments. The psychiatry consultant would also arrange with other departments for their input into psychiatry; for example, involvement of internal medicine and physiology in the psychosomatic section of the psychiatric curriculum.

The clinical psychiatry module taught in the second year is a heavy clinical experience with at least half of every day involved in diagnosis and treatment of both inpatients in hospitals and outpatients in clinics. This work should occur within a sixty-mile radius of the medical school to provide careful control by full-time staff and the presentation of didactic material that is necessary during the clinical phase. Outpatient diagnosis and treatment will be carried out in the South Plains Guidance Center and emergency rooms of the general hospitals. Inpatient diagnosis and treatment will be done in psychiatric units of affiliated general hospitals as well as the day hospital at St. Mary's Hospital. This teaching module will make use of comprehensive case studies (under supervision), methods and techniques of brief psychotherapy, field trips (state hospitals, special treatment facilities), techniques in psychopharmacology, and somatic therapies. Didactic presentations will focus on psychopathology and psychosomatic medicine and will make use of lectures, movies, tapes, and small group discussions. At the beginning of the clinical psychiatry phase an intensive course in interview techniques will be taught, making use of clinical demonstrations and televised patient interviews.

The third-year psychiatry elective lasts approximately ten weeks and is carried out on the main campus, within the sixty-mile clinical commuter campus, or in a tertiary affiliation such as Amarillo or El Paso. The following electives will be offered: (1) behavioral science; (2) behavioral science research seminar; (3) child psychiatry, including diagnostic and treatment conferences, evaluation of cases under supervision, and other teaching conferences; (4) psychotherapy; (5) psychiatric emergencies (crisis intervention); (6) psychiatric consultation; (7) community psychiatry; (8) research in psychophysiology; (9) psychosomatic medicine; (10) adolescent psychiatry; and (11) psychometrics.

Eastern Virginia

The following material outlines four integrated characteristics of a coordinated and sequential training experience in both the behavioral sciences and clinical psychiatry which are being implemented as the core of a still-to-be detailed curriculum for the Center for Behavioral Sciences.

The initial step in developing this program is to establish a well-rounded *basic* behavioral science program for the beginning medical student. This program needs to be on a par in quality and emphasis with the basic medical science program which includes physiology, biochemistry, anatomy, and so forth. For the behavioral sciences, some of these basic educational areas include the genetics of human behavior, anthropology, sociology, psychology, and human ecology. The fundamental knowledge in these areas of human experience is no longer a luxury or a curiosity, but an essential acquisition for later understanding of the dynamics of the human personality, its deviations and maladaptive forms, which the physician will deal with, whatever his medical practice. Just as anatomy is essential for the surgeon and physiology for the internist, so these disciplines are essential for an understanding of contemporary psychiatry and its unfolding directions.

A second feature of this new program for the Eastern Virginia Medical School is what we have labeled "dual teaching" of psychiatry during the later clinical years, psychiatry to be taught where possible in conjunction with the other medical specialties on the wards and in the community. That is, much of human behavior in its adaptive and maladaptive forms should be learned by the student simultaneously with learning about the individual patient seen on any of the medical or surgical wards.

For example, while making rounds, an obstetrician might demonstrate the techniques for taking a Papanicolaou smear and later describe the therapeutic techniques for treating cancer of the cervix. Making rounds at the same time would be a clinical psychiatrist, who would discuss the patient's feelings about having such an examination in front of six or seven medical students and what kind of emotional problems arise from the anxieties and fears concerned with the possibility of incurring a cancerous disease. This integrated teaching, we hope, would go a long way toward helping to produce the "compassionate scientist" that is our goal.

The third and fourth principles of this program for teaching human behavior consist of two interwoven sequences, unfolding simultaneously. The first of these sequences will proceed from learning the genetic factors in *individual* human behavior (genetics, neuroanatomy, neurophysiology), through the *environmental* factors influencing that behavior (sociology, anthropology, psychology), to studies of the *interactional* aspects of the relationship between these two (systems analysis, ethology, family dynamics). The second such sequence will be designed to encourage the flow of learning from the "normal" spectrum to the "abnormal" spectrum, from adaptive to maladaptive responses of the individual and his environment, and their interaction.

Hence, learning about the genetics of the individual, his adaptive mutations and eventually maladaptive inborn errors of metabolism, would lead to studies of environmental influences on the individual which encourage adaptation and then to examination of those which interfere with successful adaptation (sensory deprivation, maternal deprivation, and the like). A similar pattern of studying interactional dynamics, both successful and unsuccessful, would follow.

With this foundation in genetics, in the psychology of the individual and his identified environment, and in the interaction of these two, combined with a comprehension of normal personality growth and development, the student will then tackle at the end of his training period the diagnosis and treatment of minor and major psychiatric illness. By this time and by this method, his foundation should be such that these illnesses are more comprehensible, their dynamics more easily understood than they would have been without it; he can now acquire specific skills in alleviating these particular problems (as practiced with the various psychotherapies, chemotherapies, and others).

This overview and admitted simplification of the sequential learning experience will, hopefully, give one a feeling for the kind of evolution of learning experiences anticipated in the medical school years. This outline should clearly identify the need for a significant basic behavioral science program.

꧁꧁꧁꧁꧁꧁ Appendix B ꧂꧂꧂꧂꧂꧂꧂

Annotated Bibliography on Mental Health Education and List of Resources for Instructional Aids

꧁꧁꧁꧁꧁꧁꧁꧁꧁꧁꧁꧁꧂꧂꧂꧂꧂꧂꧂꧂꧂꧂꧂꧂

Books on Mental Health Education

BECKETT, P. G. S., DOMINO, E. F., AND BLEAKLEY, S. *A Teaching Program in Psychiatry*. Vol. II: *Psychoneurosis, Organic Brain Disease, Psychopharmacology*. Detroit: Wayne State Press, 1969.

The series of teaching programs is designed to permit a student to establish a basic framework of psychiatric knowledge. Subjects include the clinical content of psychoneurosis, organic brain disease, and psychopharmacology. This second volume of the two-volume series presents case material as well as frames of programmed material.

BERGER, M. M. (Ed.) *Videotape Techniques in Psychiatric Training and Treatment*. New York: Brunner/Mazel, 1970.

An excellent resource book on videotape and closed circuit television. Includes papers on the use of videotape in training, in treatment, and on technical considerations. Contains valuable bibliographies and glossaries.

230

BIBRING, G. (Ed.) *The Teaching of Dynamic Psychiatry: A Reappraisal of the Goals and Techniques in the Teaching of Psychoanalytic Psychiatry.* New York: International Universities Press, 1968.

This volume includes papers on psychoanalytic teaching in medical school and psychiatric residency programs. There are also papers on teaching physicians in the community and on teaching house staff. Many well-known psychoanalytic educators are among contributors.

Computer-Assisted Instruction in the Health Professions: Proceedings of a Conference at Harvard Medical School. Newburyport, Mass.: ENTELEK, 1970.

Papers are presented on educational requirements, preclinical education, and clinical education. The clinical education section includes papers on patient interviewing, patient management, decision-making, and case studies.

Conference on Psychiatric Education, Cornell University, 1951. *Psychiatry in Medical Education.* Washington: American Psychiatric Association, 1952.

This is a report of the 1951 Conference on Psychiatric Education organized and conducted by the American Psychiatric Association and the Association of American Medical Colleges. This is a classic in studies of psychiatric education.

Conference on Psychiatry in Medical Education. *Teaching Psychiatry in Medical School.* Washington: American Psychiatric Association, 1969.

These are the working papers of the Conference held at Atlanta, Georgia, in 1967. Topics include philosophy of goals, social climate, milieu, medical students, content, methods, participating disciplines, and resources. There were eight commissions, one on each of these topics. Each commission provides a summary report.

Conference on the Use of Computers in Medical Education, University of Oklahoma Medical Center, 1968.

The conference report includes papers on undergraduate medical education, clinical medical education, and continuing medical education as well as discussion of the use of computers in medical libraries.

Conference on Training in Child Psychiatry. *Career Training in Child*

Psychiatry. Washington, D.C.: American Psychiatric Association, 1964.

Report of a conference on the history of training in child psychiatry, providing data on the needs for training in child psychiatry and material on curriculum content as well as methods of training.

COOMBS, R. H., AND VINCENT, C. E. (Eds.) *Psychosocial Aspects of Medical Training.* Springfield, Ill.: Charles C. Thomas, 1971.

A series of papers on medical education, medical institutions, the behavioral sciences in medical education, and various predictions about the future of medical education.

Council on Medical Television. *Television in Medical Teaching and Research: A Survey and Annotated Bibliography.* Washington: Department of HEW, 1965. Superintendent of Documents Catalog #FS 5.234:34040.

This survey of the use of television in medical schools as of 1965 lists operating costs and distribution of TV installations by department. The bibliography is useful although dated.

DE KIEFFER, R. E. *Audiovisual Instruction.* New York: Center for Applied Research in Education, 1965.

This book includes pictures, charts, models, maps, and other nonprojected materials. It also gives information on movie and slide projectors and data on physical facilities as well as on research on the use of audiovisual materials in schools.

DE KIEFFER, R. E., AND COCHRAN, L. W. Manual of Audiovisual Techniques. (2nd ed.) Englewood Cliffs, N.J.: Prentice-Hall, 1955.

This is a paperback manual which has valuable basic information on boards, pictures, charts and graphs, maps, and other demonstration materials and techniques. It also has information on projected teaching materials, such as slides, filmstrips, films, and on audio and videotape recordings.

ELLIS, J. R. (Ed.) *Methods of Learning and Techniques of Teaching: Proceedings of the Second Annual Conference of the Association for the Study of Medical Education.* London: Pitman Medical Publishing Company, 1959.

The report covers such topics as incentives to learning, use of teaching aids, tutorial systems, and other papers on the student and the teacher.

GRAVES, J., AND GRAVES, V. *Second Conference on the Use of Audio-tape in Medical Teaching.* London: Chelmsford and Essex Hospital, 1967.

Conference participants were predominantly medical educators from Britain. One session is about how tape is used in academic centers, in postgraduate teaching, and by general practitioners; other sessions deal with innovations and extension of the uses of audiotape.

JONES, M. L. *Sources of Audiovisual Materials.* Washington, D.C.: U.S. Government Printing Office, 1967. Superintendent of Documents Catalog #FS 5.235.305090.

This annotated bibliography lists audiovisual materials for elementary and secondary schools. It also includes a list of general periodicals which review audiovisual materials. The directory of publishers of audiovisual materials is especially valuable.

KLINE, N. S., AND LASKA, E. (Eds.) *Computers and Electronic Devices in Psychiatry.* New York: Grune and Stratton, 1968.

A series of papers from the IV World Congress of Psychiatry; topics include the use of computers in psychiatry, implanted electrodes, evoked responses of polarization, and sleep research.

MATHIS, J. L., PIERCE, C. M., AND PISHKIN, V. *Basic Psychiatry: A Primer of Concepts and Terminology.* New York: Appleton-Century-Crofts, 1968.

This is a programmed text for learning basic psychiatry. Part I is composed of selected definitions and terms, Part II is an outline of basic psychiatry, and Part III is a program based on the outline of Part II.

MENNINGER, K. A. *A Guide to Psychiatric Books with Some Suggested Reading Lists.* (2nd rev. ed.) New York: Grune and Stratton, 1956.

Although this volume is more than fifteen years old, it continues to have relevance as a source of many standard books in psychiatry.

Rochester Conference on Programmed Instruction in Medical Education. *Programmed Instruction in Medical Education.* Rochester: Rochester Clearinghouse, 1965.

This report of the First Rochester Conference includes studies on medical program development, on research and evaluation in programmed instruction, and on specific problems in medical programming.

Rochester Conference on Self-Instruction and Medical Education. *Self-Instruction and Medical Education.* Rochester: Rochester Clearinghouse, 1967.

These proceedings of the Second Rochester Conference on Self-Instruction include papers on the process of analyzing program material, research on self-instructional methods, and various applications of self-instruction. It attempts to go beyond the single topic of programmed instruction and gets into the entire area of self-instructional aids and procedures.

TAUBER, M., STEPHENS, F., ROEMER, I., AND OTHERS. *Conference on the Use of Printed and Audiovisual Material for Instructional Purposes.* New York: Columbia University Press, 1965.

Reviews the use of printed and audiovisual materials for instruction at the elementary, secondary, and college, and university levels. The report includes a wide bibliography on the topic, deals with information-retrieval systems, and provides instruction in library use by students.

UNWIN, D. Media and Methods Instructional Technology in Higher Education. London: McGraw-Hill, 1969.

This book includes a series of papers on audiovisual equipment and methods, programmed learning, television, instructional technology, and systems approaches, and provides data on spaces for learning and teaching.

WERKMAN, S. L. *The Role of Psychiatry in Medical Education: An Appraisal and a Forecast.* Cambridge: Harvard University Press, 1966.

Reviews issues in psychiatric education and attempts to develop the "ideal" curriculum. The book is an excellent resource for all psychiatric educators and summarizes many of the issues with great clarity.

World Health Organization. *Medical Education: Annotated Bibliography 1946–1955.* Geneva: World Health Organization, 1958.

A bibliographic listing taken from the Index Medicus and the indices and catalogs of the World Health Organization Library.

Journals on Instructional Media and Aids

AV Communication Review. Published quarterly by the Department of Audio Visual Instruction, National Education Association, 1201 Sixteenth Street N.W., Washington, D.C. 20036.

It has a number of reviews and articles and information on putting together instructional aids.

Audio Visual Instruction. Official publication of the Association for Educational Communications in Technology, 1201 Sixteenth Street N.W. Washington, D.C. 20036.

It is published ten times a year, monthly September through May with a combined June and July issue. Volume 16 (1971) has a variety of articles on audiovisual material including advertisements and other source and resource information.

Audio Visual Media International Review. The quarterly Journal of the International Council for Advancement of Audio Visual Media in Education, c/o Pergamon Press, Headington Hill Hall, Oxford OX 3 OBW England.

Theoretical articles and a practical list of films and instructional aids.

Journal of Educational Technology. Published three times a year for the National Council for Educational Technology, Councils and Educaton Press, 10 Queen Anne Street, London W1N 9LD England.

A lot of theoretical papers but also a lot of practical material.

Catalogues of Films and Other Instructional Aids

American Hospital Assn. American Hospital Association Film Library Catalogue. Contains listing of films and filmstrips which may be rented or purchased, together with suggestions for hospital education programs.

Write to: American Hospital Association
840 N. Lakeshore Dr.
Chicago, Ill. 60611

American Personnel and Guidance Assn. Catalogue of films on careers in health sciences and on process in counseling programs.

Write to: Film Dept.
American Personnel and Guidance Assn.
1607 New Hampshire Ave., N.W.
Washington, D.C. 20009

American Medical Assn. Films for professional and lay groups.
Write to: American Medical Assn.
Medical Motion Pictures and Television Section
535 N. Dearborn St.
Chicago, Ill. 60610

American Psychiatric Assn. Films available through Hospital and
Community Psychiatry Service.
Write to: American Psychiatric Association
1700 18th St., N.W.
Washington, D.C. 20009

Alabama Dept. of Public Health. Publication "Promoting Mental
Health through Educational Television."
Write to: Division of Mental Hygiene
Auburn University Educational Television
Auburn, Ala. 36830

Ciba. Catalogue of scientific information services—publications, films,
slides, and exhibits.
Write to: Ciba Pharmaceutical Company
P.O. Box 195
Summit, N.J. 07901

California Dept. of Mental Hygiene. Film catalogue including films
available from their film library.
Write to: Bureau of Mental Health Education
Dept. of Mental Hygiene
744 P St.
Sacramento, Calif. 95814

University of California. Extensive catalogue of training films.
Write to: Extension Media Center, University Extension
Berkeley, Calif. 94720

Ealing. Catalogue of film loops for colleges and universities. Includes
information on 8 mm silent film loops, equipment, and utilization techniques.
Write to: Ealing Film-Loops
2225 Massachusetts Ave.
Cambridge, Mass. 02140

Geigy. List of free films on medical education.
    Write to: Local Geigy representative

Great Plains National. Films and television tapes produced by Univ. of Nebraska.
    Write to: Great Plains National Instructional
              Television Library
              Box 80669
              Lincoln, Neb. 68501

Harper & Row. Films and film loops for colleges; other audiovisual materials.
    Write to: College Department
              Harper & Row
              49 E. 33rd St.
              New York, N.Y. 10016

Harvard. Mental health training films and film guides and other resource lists.
    Write to: Edward A. Mason, M.D.
              Laboratory of Community Psychiatry
              Dept. of Psychiatry
              33 Fenwood Rd.
              Boston, Mass. 02115

International Film Bureau. Catalogue of films, filmstrips, and equipment.
    Write to: International Film Bureau
              332 S. Michigan Ave.
              Chicago, Ill. 60604

Lilly. Films, slides, and pamphlets.
    Write to: Eli Lilly & Co.
              P.O. Box 814
              Indianapolis, Ind. 46206

Medcom. Variety of audiovisual resources.
    Write to: Medcom, Inc.
              280 Park Ave.
              New York, N.Y. 10017

Mississippi. Publication on television and videotape in psychiatry and bibliography.
Write to: Floy Jack Moore, M.D.
        Univ. of Mississippi Medical Center
        Jackson, Miss. 36755

Michigan. Joint Michigan State, Univ. of Michigan Film Catalogue.
Write to: University of Michigan Audio-Visual Center
        Ann Arbor, Michigan 48104

National Clearinghouse for Mental Health Information. Films, resources, distributors, and other directories. PHS Publication 1591.
Write to: National Clearinghouse for
        Mental Health Information
        National Institute of Mental Health
        5600 Fishers Lane
        Rockville, Maryland 20852

Merrell. Medical films.
Write to: Wm. S. Merrell Co.
        1269 Gest St.
        Cincinnati, Ohio 45203

Mountain Plains Educational Media Council. Extensive and complete catalogue of training films.
Write to: Bureau of Audio-visual Instruction
        University of Colorado
        Boulder, Colo. 80304

Multi-Media Resource Center. Films, tapes, and other educational materials on human sexuality.
Write to: Multi-Media Resource Center
        340 Jones St., Box 439
        San Francisco, Calif. 94102

Network for Continuing Medical Education. Television programs for health professionals.
Write to: Network for Continuing Medical Education
        342 Madison Ave.
        New York, N.Y. 10017

National Medical Audiovisual Center. Mental health film guide, semi-

nars/workshops, other services including videotapes.
Write to: National Medical Audiovisual Center
1600 Clifton Rd. N.E.
Atlanta, Ga. 30333

Oklahoma. "Films in the Behavioral Sciences; An Annotated Catalogue," by J. M. Schneider, B. Addis, and M. Addis. 2nd ed. Behavioral Sciences Media Laboratory.
Write to: Behavioral Sciences Media Laboratory
Dept. of Psychiatry and Behavioral Sciences
Univ. of Oklahoma Medical Center
Oklahoma City, Okla. 73104

Pennsylvania State University. Psychological cinema register—films in the behavioral sciences.
Write to: Audio-Visual Services
Pennsylvania State University
University Park, Pa. 16802

Pfizer. Medical education films.
Write to: Pfizer Laboratories Film Library
267 W. 25th St.
New York, N.Y. 10001

Sandoz. Medical films.
Write to: Film Department
Sandoz Pharmaceuticals
East Hanover, N.J. 07936

Scott and White Clinic. Psychiatric films and videotapes produced by Dr. Harry Wilmer.
Write to: Dept. of Psychiatry
Scott and White Clinic
Temple, Texas 75601

Smith Kline & French. Films, pamphlets, medical television, and other services.
Write to: Smith Kline & French Laboratories
1500 Spring Garden St.
Philadelphia, Pa. 19101

Squibb. Medical motion pictures.
Write to: Squibb
745 Fifth Ave.
New York, N.Y. 10022

US Army. Army films for civilian and professional medical groups.
     Write to: Sixth US Army Central Audio-Visual Support Center
               Bldg. 603
               Presidio of San Francisco, Calif. 94129

Bibliography

American Psychiatric Association. *Psychiatry and Medical Education. Report of 1951, Ithaca Conference.* Washington, D.C., 1952.

American Psychiatric Association. *The Psychiatrist, His Training and Development. Report of the 1952 Ithaca Conference.* Washington, D.C., 1953.

American Psychiatric Association. *Teaching Psychiatry in Medical Schools: Working Papers of the Conference on Psychiatry and Medical Education, 1967.* Washington, D.C., 1969.

AVNET, H. H. *Psychiatric Insurance.* New York: Group Health Insurance, 1962.

AVNET, H. H. "Psychiatric Insurance: Ten Years Later." *American Journal of Psychiatry,* 1969, *126,* 667–674.

BARROWS, H. S. *Simulated Patients (Programmed Patients); The Development and Use of a New Technique in Medical Education.* Springfield, Ill.: Thomas, 1971.

BARROWS, H. S., AND ABRAHAMSON, S. "The Programmed Patient: A Technique for Appraising Student Performance in Clinical Neurology." *Journal of Medical Education,* 1964, *39,* 802–805.

BEAUMONT, G., FEIGAL, D., AND MAGRAW, R. M. "Medical Auditing in a

241

Comprehensive Clinical Program." *Journal of Medical Education*, 1967, *42*, 359–367.

Carnegie Commission on Higher Education. *Higher Education and the Nation's Health: Policies for Medical and Dental Education: A Special Report and Recommendations*. New York: McGraw-Hill, 1970.

CHARVAT, J., MC GUIRE, C., AND PARSONS, V. *A Review of the Nature and Uses of Examinations in Medical Education*. New York: American Public Health Association, 1968, 74 pages.

COLBY, K. M., WATT, J. B., AND GILBERT, J. P. "A Computer Method of Psychotherapy: A Preliminary Communication." *Journal of Nervous and Mental Disorders*, 1966, *142*, 148–152.

COLMORE, J. P. "Evaluation of Daily Student Performance." *Journal of American Medical Association*, 1966, *198*, 293–295.

CUMMING, N., AND FOLLETT, W. T. "Psychiatric Services and Medical Utilization in a Prepaid Health Plan Setting, Part 2." *Medical Care*, 1968, *6*, 31–41.

DONABEDIAN, A. "Evaluating the Quality of Medical Care." *Milbank Memorial Fund Quarterly*, 1966, *44*, 166–203.

EARLEY, L. W. (Ed.) *Teaching Psychiatry in Medical School*. Washington, D.C.: American Psychiatric Association, 1969.

EBAUGH, F. G. "The History of Psychiatric Education in the United States from 1844–1944." *American Journal of Psychiatry*, 1944, *100*, 151–161.

EBAUGH, F. G., AND RYMER, C. A. Psychiatry in Medical Education. New York: The Commonwealth Fund, 1942.

ENELOW, A. J., ADLER, L. M., AND WEXLER, M. "Programmed Instruction in Interviewing: An Experiment in Medical Education." *Journal of the American Medical Association*, 1970, *212*, 1843–1846.

FEIN, R., AND WEBER, G. I. *Financing Medical Education*. New York: McGraw-Hill, 1971.

FOLIMAN, J. F., JR. *Insurance Coverage for Mental Illness*. New York: American Management Association, 1970.

GLASSER, M. A. "Mental Health, National Health Insurance, and the Economy." *Hospital and Community Psychiatry*, 1972, *23*, 17–22.

GOLDENSOHN, S. S., FINK, R., AND SHAPIRO, S. *APA Guidelines for Psychiatric Services Covered Under Health Insurance Plans*. 2nd ed. Washington, D.C.: American Psychiatric Association, 1969a.

GOLDENSOHN, S. S., FINK, R., AND SHAPIRO, S. *1969 Source Book of Health Insurance Data.* New York: Health Insurance Institute, 1969b.

GOLDENSOHN, S. S., FINK, R., AND SHAPIRO, S. "Referral, Utilization, and Staffing Patterns of a Mental Health Service in a Prepaid Group Practice Program in New York." *American Journal of Psychiatry,* November 1969c, *126,* 689–698.

GONNELLA, J. S. "Evaluation of Patient Care, An Approach." *Journal of the American Medical Association,* 1970, *214,* 2040-2043.

GOLDBERG, I. D., KRANTZ, G., AND LOCKE, B. Z. "Effect of a Short-Term Outpatient Psychiatric Therapy Benefit on the Utilization of Medical Services in a Prepaid Group Practice Medical Program." *Medical Care,* 1970, *8,* 419–428.

GRAVES, W. W. "Some Factors Tending Toward Adequate Instruction in Nervous and Mental Disease." *Journal of the American Medical Association,* 1914, *63,* 1707–1713.

Group for the Advancement of Psychiatry. Report No. 54. *The Preclinical Teaching of Psychiatry.* New York, 1962.

HAMBURG, D. A. (Ed.) *Psychiatry As a Behavioral Science.* Englewood Cliffs, N.J.: Prentice Hall, 1961.

HARLESS, W. G., AND OTHERS. "CASE: A Computer-Aided Simulation of the Clinical Encounter." *Journal of Medical Education,* 1971, *46,* 443–448.

HELFER, R. E. "An Objective Comparison of the Pediatric Interviewing Skills of Freshman and Senior Medical Students." *Pediatrics,* 1970, *45,* 623–627.

HELFER, R. E., AND HESS, J. "An Experimental Model for Making Objective Measurements of Interviewing Skills." *Journal of Clinical Psychology,* 1970, *26,* 327–331.

HUBBARD, J. P. *Measuring Medical Education: The Tests and Test Procedures of the National Board of Medical Examiners.* Philadelphia: Lea and Febiger, 1971.

JASON, H. "The Current and Potential Use of Course Examinations." *Journal of the American Medical Association,* 1966, *198,* 289–290.

LANGSLEY, D. G. "Training and Service: Flirtation, Affair or Marriage?" Paper delivered at Conference on Residency Training in Community Mental Health Centers, Aspen, Colorado, June 8, 1972.

LEIGHTON, A. H. "The Other Side of the Coin." *Hospital Tribune and Medical News,* 1971, *5,* 11.

LEMBCKE, P. A. "Evolution of the Medical Audit." *Journal of the American Medical Association,* 1967, *199,* 543–550.

LEVINE, H. G., AND MC GUIRE, C. H. "Role-Playing As an Evaluation Technique." *Journal of Educational Measurement,* 1968, *5,* 1–8.

LEVIT, E. J. "The Use of Motion Pictures in Testing the Clinical Competence of Physicians." *Annals of the New York Academy of Sciences,* 1967, *142,* 449–454.

MOREHEAD, M. A. "The Medical Audit As an Operational Tool." *American Journal of Public Health,* 1967, *57,* 1643–1656.

MYERS, E. S. "Insurance Coverage for Mental Illness: Present Status and Future Prospects." *American Journal of Public Health,* 1970, *60,* 1921–1930.

MYERS, E. S. "Coverage of Mental Disorders under Insurance Plans." Presented at the Annual Conference of State Mental Health Representatives, American Medical Association, Chicago, September 1971. Available on request from the American Psychiatric Association, Washington, D.C.

National Academy of Sciences. *The Behavioral and Social Sciences: Outlook and Needs.* Englewood Cliffs, N.J.: Prentice Hall, 1969.

NOBLE, R. A. *Psychiatry in Medical Education.* New York: National Committee for Mental Hygiene, 1933.

NURNBERGER, J. I. "The Brief for the Inclusion of Relevant Contributions from the Basic Biological Sciences Within the Broad Spectrum of Behavioral Sciences." In L. W. Earley, *Teaching Psychiatry in Medical School.* Washington, D.C.: American Psychiatric Association, 1969.

PRICE, P. B., TAYLOR, C. W., AND RICHARDS, J. M., JR. "Measurement of Physician Performance." *Journal of Medical Education,* 1964, *39,* 203–210.

REED, L. S. "Private Health Insurance, 1968: Enrollment, Coverage and Financial Experience." *Social Security Bulletin,* 1969, *32,* 3–19.

REED, L. S., MYERS, E. S., AND SCHEIDEMANDEL, P. L. *Insurance Plans and Patient Care: Utilization and Costs.* Washington, D.C.: American Psychiatric Association, 1972.

ROMANO, J. "Requiem or Reveille: The Clinician's Choice." *Journal of Medical Education,* 1963, *38,* 584–590.

ROMANO, J. "And Leave for the Unknown." *Journal of the American Medical Association,* 1964, *190,* 282–284.

ROMANO, J. "Teaching Medical Students about Population, Sexual

Practices, and Family Planning." *The Journal of Medical Education,* 1968, *43,* 898–906.

ROMANO, J. "The Teaching of Psychiatry to Medical Students: Past, Present, and Future." *American Journal of Psychiatry,* 1970a, *126,* 1115–1126.

ROMANO, J. "The Elimination of the Internship—An Act of Regression." *American Journal of Psychiatry,* 1970b, *126,* 1565–1576.

ROMANO, J. "Current Trends in Undergraduate and Graduate Medical Teaching." *Journal of Nervous and Mental Disease,* 1972, *154,* 186–192.

SCHEIDEMANDEL, P., KANNO, C., AND GLASSCOTE, R. *Health Insurance for Mental Illness.* Washington, D.C.: Joint Information Service, American Psychiatric Association, 1967.

SCOTT, N. C., JR., GALLAGHER, R. E., AND HESS, J. W. "Interaction Analysis As a Method for Assessing Interviewing Behavior." *Journal of Medical Education,* 1970, *45,* 815.

SIMMONS, L. W., AND BROSIN, H. W. "The Role of Social and Behavioral Scientists in the Present and Possible Future Functions of the Medical School, Especially in Departments of Psychiatry." In L. W. Earley, *Teaching Psychiatry in Medical School.* Washington, D.C.: American Psychiatric Association, 1969.

STEVENS, R. *American Medicine and the Public Interest.* New Haven, Conn.: Yale University Press, 1971.

STOKES, J. F. "Examining in the United States: The National Board of Medical Examiners." *British Journal of Medical Education,* 1967, *1,* 320–329.

STRAUS, R. "Behavioral Science in the Medical Curriculum." *Annals of the New York Academy of Sciences,* 1965, *128,* 599–606.

TEMPLETON, B. *Chart Audit Evaluation of Application of Psychiatric Skills in Non-Psychiatric Setting.* Thesis, Degree of Master of Education, University of Illinois, 1969.

VON MERING, O. "Behavioral Sciences in Medical and Psychiatric Education with Special Reference to Anthropology and Sociology." In L. W. Earley, *Teaching Psychiatry in Medical School.* Washington, D.C.: American Psychiatric Association, 1969.

WARE, J. E., JR., STRASSMAN, H. D., AND NAFTULIN, D. H. "A Negative Relationship Between Understanding Interviewing Principles and Interview Performance." *Journal of Medical Education,* 1971, *46,* 620–622.

WEBSTER, T. G. "Psychiatry and Behavioral Science Curriculum Time in U.S. Schools of Medicine and Osteopathy." *Journal of Medical Education,* 1967, *42,* 687–696.

WEED, L. L. *Medical Records, Medical Education, and Patient Care.* Cleveland: Press of Case Western Reserve University, 1969.

WILLIAMSON, J. W., ALEXANDER, M., AND MILLER, G. E. "Continuing Education and Patient Care Research." *Journal of American Medical Association,* 1967, *201,* 938–942.

WOMACK, N. A. "The Evolution of the National Board of Medical Examiners." *Journal of the American Medical Association,* 1965, *192,* 817–823.

World Health Organization. *The Undergraduate Teaching of Psychiatry and Mental Health Promotion, Ninth Report of the Expert Committee on Mental Health.* Technical Report Series No. 208, Geneva, 1961.

ZIMET, C. N. "Clinical Psychology in Undergraduate Medical Education." In L. W. Earley, *Teaching Psychiatry in Medical School.* Washington, D.C.: American Psychiatric Association, 1969.

Index

A

ADSETT, A., 1–2, 3–18, 30
Aetna Insurance Company, 134
Airlie House Conference. *See* Conference on Mental Health Education in New Medical Schools
American Board of Psychiatry and Neurology, 36, 217
American Medical Association, 128–129, 181
American Psychiatric Association, 127–128, 130, 141–142
American River College, 77
A.P.A.-N.A.M.H. Joint Information Service, 128
Arizona Medical Center, 164
Assessment. *See* Evaluation
Association of American Medical Colleges, 63
AVNET, H. H, 127

B

BARROWS, H. S., 93
BARTON, W. E., 127–139, 141–142

BEAUMONT, G., 94
Behavioral objectives. *See* Objectives, behavioral
Behavioral science: definition of, 19–28, 159; future role of, 159–160; goals of, 21–22; integration of in McMaster experience, 8–9; integration of in other departments, 24, 159; justification for in medical school, 25–26, 33; as separate department, 2, 21–22, 24–25, 32–33, 159–160; status of teacher of, 23, 32; titles for departments of, 25. *See also* specific schools
BERTSCH, E. F., 19
Beth Israel Hospital, 199
Bexar County Teaching Hospital, 222
BISHOP, F. M., 19, 25
BLAIN, D., 128
Blue Cross–Blue Shield, 131, 133
BROSIN, H. W., 25
Brown University, 164–168

C

Canadian health insurance programs, 131, 135, 142
CARROLL, L., 25
CHAMPUS Program, 125, 136
CHARVAT, J., 88–89
Child psychiatry: in psychiatric residency training, 51. *See also* specific schools
City University of New York, 200
CLEGHORN, J., 8
Clinical clerkships, 151–152; in McMaster program, 5, 16. *See also* specific schools
Clinical settings: definition of, 59–60. *See also* Settings for educational programs; specific schools
COHEN, R., 47
COLBY, K. M., 97
COLMORE, J. P., 91
Commonwealth Fund, Conference on Psychiatric Education of, 63
Communities served by psychiatric residency trainees. *See* Psychiatry residency training
Community mental health center model, 154–156, 161–162; combined with other health care services, 154; problems of as medical school training setting, 155; use of interdisciplinary team in, 154. *See also* specific schools
Community psychiatry, 110–112
Competency objectives. *See* Objectives, behavioral
Confederate Memorial Center, 189
Conference on Mental Health Education in New Medical Schools, 149
Conference on Psychiatric Education of the Commonwealth Fund, 63
Conference on Psychiatry and Medical Education, 25
Congress, U.S.: funding of training programs by, 114; insurance

bills proposed by, 117, 136–137
Construction, capital, 153
Continuing education, 40, 51–52, 155, 162
Continuing Education Branch, NIMH, 57–58
Core curriculum, 47–48, 50, 55, 71. *See also* specific schools
Crisis intervention: training in, 27, 45; types of problems encountered in, 75–76
CUMMING, N., 143

D

Delivery, health care: dissatisfaction with, 147–148; psychiatry's role in, 153; trends in systems of, 139–141, 153, 160–162
Departmental clerkships: as opposed to general clerkships, 151–152
Diagnostic skills, 102–103
Disadvantaged students. *See* Minorities and ethnic subcultures
DONABEDIAN, A., 94
Drew Postgraduate Medical School, 177–178

E

Eastern Virginia Medical School, 66–67, 227–229; role of psychiatry at, 228–229; and sequential learning experience as core curriculum for Center for Behavioral Sciences, 227–229
EBAUGH, F. G., 63
Electives: in residency training, 47–48. *See also* specific schools
Elmhurst Hospital, 199
Enabling objectives, 81–83
ENELOW, A. J., 52, 91; identification of nine types of psychiatrists by, 52
Evaluation: of educational objectives, 66, 162; of National Health Insurance Plans, 123–125, 162. *See also* Evaluation of student performance; Objectives, behavioral

Evaluation of student performance, 88–98; by audit of medical record entries, 93–98; competency objectives for, 101–112; computer simulations in, 97–98; exams for, 88–92, 97, 99; films for, 90–92; human simulations for, 92–93, 97; by National Board, 90; reliability of, 88, 90–92, 100; by residents, 100; with taped student-patient interactions, 93–98; use of machine scoring and data processing in, 89–90, 97; use of recorded material in, 96–97; "validity" of defined, 91

Examinations, 88–92, 97, 99

F

Faculty, new activities of medical, 148

Family physicians, upgrading of, 16–17

Federal employees' benefit insurance program, 131, 141–142

FELIX, R., 21

FLETCHER, R., 25

FOLEY, H. A., 115–126

FOLLETTE, W. T., 143

Funding, 45–46, 54–55, 113–145, 155, 160–162; annual cost of, 115; availability of, 115–116; of construction, 153; evaluating mechanisms of, 117–118; by NIMH, 54–55, 114; of psychiatric residency training under support of H.M.O. and third-party payment, 45–46, 55, 137–138; reduction of, 114, 137; through research 114, 160; various means of, 118. *See also* Insurance, commercial; National Health Insurance Program

G

Genesee County Community Mental Health Services, 192

GIRSHMAN, K., 129

GLASSCOTE, R., 128

GLASSER, M. A., 128–130

GOLDBERG, I. D., 143

GONNELLA, J. S., 91

GRAVES, W. W., 63

Group for the Advancement of Psychiatry, 19

Group Health Insurance, Inc., 127, 130, 143

Guidelines for competency objectives, 101–112

H

HAMBURG, D. A., 20

HARLESS, W. G., 97

HARRELL, G. T., 25

Harvard School of Public Health, 49

Health care delivery. *See* Delivery, health care

Health Maintenance Organization, 73, 142–144, 160–162; and community mental health center, 144; psychiatric residency training support under, 45–46, 55. *See also* National Health Insurance Program

HELFER, R. E., 93

HESS, J. W., 93

Hill-Burton funds, 153

H.M.O. *See* Health Maintenance Organization

HUBBARD, J. P., 89

Human services, emphasis on, 148

I

Impact tendencies for National Health Insurance Program, 119–123

Instructional objectives, 79–87

Insurance, commercial, 118, 131–134

Interdisciplinary training. *See* Multidisciplinary education

Internship: abolishment of, 39, 46, 60, 154, 156–157; rotating, 13

Interviewing skills, 103–105

Ithaca Conference on Psychiatric Education, 63–64

J

JASON, H., 77, 79–87, 89, 93, 99–
    100, 190
Johns Hopkins, 24, 130
Joint Commission on Accreditation
    of Hospitals, 134, 136

K

Kaiser–Permanente Plan, 10, 131,
    135, 142–144
KANNO, C., 128
Kauikeolani Children's Hospital, 185
KRANTZ, G., 143

L

LANGSLEY, D. G., 147–162
Law, psychiatry and the, 107–108
LEIGHTON, A. H., 49
LEMBCKE, P. A., 94
LEVINE, H. G., 93
LEVIT, E. J., 90
Licensure, 89–90, 93
LOCKE, B. Z., 143
Louisiana State University–Shreve-
    port, 188–189

M

McMaster University, 1–18, 30–31,
    150; administrative organiza-
    tion of, 5, 6; alliance of psy-
    chiatry with family medicine
    at, 15–18; clinical clerkship
    in, 5, 16–18; educational ob-
    jectives of, 6–11; electives in,
    4, 12–14; goals of undergrad-
    uate psychiatric education of,
    14–15; horizontal programs of,
    4; integration of basic sciences
    with clinical medicine at, 8;
    integration of other disciplines
    at, 8–11; length of training at,
    4–5, 13; medical education as
    a whole in, 13; phases of, 4–7,
    12; primary health care teams
    in, 17; residency training in,
    13; responsibilities of faculty
    of, 6, 9–14; role of psychiatry
    in, 14–18; student participa-
    tion in organization of, 5; tu-

torial system of, 4, 11–14, 31.
    See also Matrix management
    model
MC PARTLAND, T., 129
MAGER, B., 81
MANDELL, A. F., 9
Matrix management model, 3, 5; def-
    inition of, 5–6, 30; at McMas-
    ter, 1–18, 30–31; problems of,
    6, 31
Medicaid, 125–126
Medical College of Ohio, at Toledo,
    66, 209–210
Medical education: changes in, 1–2,
    156–157; goal of, 82, 161;
    length of, 156–157; systems
    analysis approach to, 37. *See
    also* specific schools; Intern-
    ship; McMaster University;
    Psychiatric education
Medical school departments, creation
    of, 21–24
Medical schools as trainees for all
    health professions, 148
Medicare, 125–126, 129, 135
Mental health care: cost of annually,
    133–136; number of patients
    served by, 132–136. *See also*
    National Health Insurance
    Program
Mental status examination, 81–82
MEYER, A., 20
Michigan Health and Social Security
    Research Institute, 128–130
Michigan State University, 24, 68,
    99, 155, 189–193; community
    involvement of, 190; integra-
    tion of College of Human
    Medicine with, 189–190; med-
    ical student education at, 191–
    192; psychiatry clerkships at,
    190; research and education
    in health services at, 190–191;
    research in medical education
    at, 190–191; residency train-
    ing at, 192–193
MILLER, P. R., 174
Minorities and ethnic subcultures:
    education of, 100; profession-

als of, 145, 158; recruitment of, 100, 158, 162; responsibility of medical schools to, 157–159, 162; students of, 158–159; teaching about problems of, 41

MOREHEAD, M. A., 94

Mount Sinai, 199–202; curriculum of school of medicine at, 199–202; establishment of school of medicine at, 199; objectives of department of psychiatry of, 200–202; residency program at, 201–202

Multidisciplinary education: 1–2, 40; by committee, 2; future of, 150–152; group planning of, 5; integration of departments in, 9; problems of, 6, 40–41; in psychiatric residency training, 48, 53–55, 67–68, 71, 75–76; team approach to, 119–120, 124–125, 140; at University of Missouri (Kansas City), 31; various clinical settings in, 15–16. *See also* McMaster University

MYERS, E. S., 131

N

National Academy of Sciences, report of, 20

National Association for Mental Health, 127

National Association of Private Psychiatric Hospitals, 128

National Association of State Mental Health Program Directors, 128

National Board of Medical Examiners, 88–90, 101

National Health Care System. *See* National Health Insurance Program

National Health Insurance Program, 113–114, 116–145, 161–162; assessment and evaluation of, 123–125; and Blue Cross-Blue Shield plan, 131, 133, 142; Canadian experience in, 131, 135, 142; and CHAMPUS program, 125, 135; and commercial insurance, 131, 133–135; cost of mental health care, under, 133–136, 142–143; coverage of, 118, 132–136; criteria for optimal mental health coverage under, 123–125, 141; desirable plan for, 116, 118–126; feasibility of, 127; and federal employees' benefit insurance program, 131; impact of on educational programs, 137–138, 161; impact of on services, 136–138; and Kaiser-Permanente plan, 131, 135, 142–144; N.I.M.H. Task Force on, 123; number of days of coverage by, 130–131, 133–134; Reed Report on, 142–143; states with mental health coverage in, 142; U.A.W. plan for, 129–131, 136; workshop on psychiatric issues of, 128

National Institute of Mental Health, 21, 36, 40, 42, 48, 54–55, 58, 66, 114, 123, 128, 133, 144, 184

National Institutes of Health, 21

New medical schools: interdepartmental curricula in, 150–152; settings of, 57, 65, 73, 152–156; under development, 150–152

NIXON, R. M., 119, 144

NOBLE, R. A., 63

North Oakland Community Mental Health Center, 192

NURNBERGER, J. I., 19

O

Objectives, behavioral (competency, performance), 77–112; for complex and subtle activities, 83–84; for courses, 84–85; criteria for writing, 85–86; definition of, 81–82; for different years or phases, 84–85; enabling, 82–83; evaluating achievement of, 77–78, 85–86; for first-year training, 78; guidelines for, 78, 101–112; identifying areas requiring, 84, 99–100; need for, 80–81; priorities for setting, 77–87, 101; questions asked before writing, 79–87; as restraints, 86–87; specificity of, 83–84; terminal, 82–83

Office of Management and Budget, 137

P

Pacific Medical Center, 101

PELLEGRINO, E., 27

Pennsylvania State University at Hershey, 25, 66, 210–213; general consultation and education at, 213; graduate student education at, 211; psychiatric residency training at, 211–213; role of department of psychiatry at, 210–213

PFEILLER, R., 129

Planning psychiatric training, 77–112; mastery model for, 77, 100–101. *See also* Evaluation of student performance; Objectives, behavioral

Pontiac State Hospital, 192

Premedical studies, 156; relevance of, 100

Preventive psychiatry, 17, 45–46, 55, 121, 140, 147

PRICE, P. B., 91

Primary care physicians: definition of, 16; lack of contact with students by, 152; in McMaster program, 16. *See also* Family physicians

Professional growth, 108–109

Program descriptions of mental health education in new medical schools. *See* specific schools

Psychiatric education: basic sciences in, 1; changes in, 1–2; goals of, 3, 14–18; interdisciplinary teaching vs. traditional depart-

mental, 1–2; length of, 156–157; at McMaster University, 1–18; matrix management model of, 1–18; methods of achieving goals in, 3; role of psychiatry department in, 1–2; undergraduate, 14–18. *See also* Psychiatry residency training; specific schools

Psychiatrists, types of, 52

Psychiatry: communities served by, 42; definition of, 20–21; effect of loss of internship on, 46; students of, 23; validity of the old modes of, 43

Psychiatry department: basic sciences in, 1; definition of, 20–21, 149; divisions within, 28; interdisciplinary teaching by, 1–2; in McMaster program, 8

Psychiatry residency training, 35–55; in alcoholism treatment, 51; assessment of, 39, 41; career choice of during, 39, 52, 157; changes needed in, 42–49, 51–55; in child psychiatry, 51; for community service, 42–49; community to be served by, 42–46, 51–55, 57–76; core curriculum in, 47–48, 50, 55; critical mass problem in, 53–54; in drug abuse treatment, 51; electives in, 47–48, 50; funding of, 45–46, 54–55; goals of, 37–38, 40, 42–48, 51–52; as influenced by age of medical school, 38; interdisciplinary, 48, 50, 52–54; makeup of typical block program in, 38–39, 44–45; in neurology, 41, 51; program planning approach to, 38; psychoanalytic, 41, 46–47, 51; in research, 48; responsibilities of director of, 44–45, 72; rotation in, 35, 41; settings for, 38, 40, 43–45, 50; supported by H.M.O. and third-party payment systems, 45–46, 55; teaching about minorities and their problems in, 41, 45, 51, 76; track system in, 47–48, 50. *See also* Objectives, behavioral; specific schools

Psychiatry Training Branch, NIMH, 36, 48–49

Psychoanalytic training, 41, 46–47, 51

R

REED, L. S., 118, 131, 142

Research: funding of, 114, 148, 160; training for, 48

Residency training. *See* Psychiatry residency training

RESNIK, H. L. P., 2, 19–29, 32, 159

ROMANO, J., 57, 59–64

Roosevelt University, 130

Rotating internship, 13

Rush-Presbyterian St. Luke's Medical Center, 213–219; child psychiatry training program at, 218–219; graduate psychiatry at, 217–218; objectives of psychiatry courses at, 215–216; required courses at, 216–217; undergraduate program at, 213–215

RYMER, C., 63

S

Sacramento State College, 177

SAID, 169, 174

St. Joseph's Hospital, 180

St. Mary's Hospital, 227

St. Vincent Hospital, 210

San Antonio Children's Center, 222

SCHEIDEMANDEL, P. L., 128, 131

SCOTT, N. C., JR., 92

Settings for educational programs, 56–57, 152–156; catchment area concept of, 57, 61–63, 65, 71–72, 74–75, 154–155; clinical, 59–64; control of services and education in, 72–74; criteria for determining optimal, 59–60, 65–70, 72–76; definition of clinical, 59–60; design of for patient care, 69; evaluation of, 66–68, 153; goals of, 59–60, 65–70, 72–76; influences of on programs, 60–68, 71–72; programs developed before, 66; scope of education student must experience in, 60–64, 69, 74–75; as set up by new schools, 57, 65, 73, 159; small inpatient hospital, 57, 61–64, 71, 152; supervision in, 63–64, 75; use of interdisciplinary training in, 67–68, 71, 75–76; variety of patient experience in, 61–64, 69, 74–75

SHAKOW, D., 61

SHERVINGTON, W. W., 36, 42–50

SIMMONS, L. W., 25

Slide tapes, 8

SMITH, S., 8

Social Science Research Council, 1969 report of, 20

Southern Illinois University, 186–188

Southwestern Medical School at Dallas, 36

Specialty Board Certification, 89, 93

Specialty training programs, length of, 157

STAINBROOK, E., 24

State University of New York at Stony Brook, 67, 155, 205–209; curriculum of, 205; educational program in department of psychiatry at, 206–209; instructional goals at, 207–209; role of basic sciences and role of clinical sciences at, 205

STOKES, J. F., 89

STRAUS, R., 21–22, 25

STUBBLEFIELD, R. L., 35–41, 50

Suicide prevention, 27

Systems analysis approach, definition of, 37

Systems Analysis Index for Diagnosis of Basic Psychiatric Syndromes Handbook, 169, 174

T

Tampa General Hospital, 180–181

Teaching aids, 230–240
Temple University, 24
TEMPLETON, B., 78, 88–98, 100
Terminal objectives, 82–83
Texas Tech University, 223–227;
  general medical school program at, 223–226; psychiatry
  curriculum details at, 226–
  227; role of department of
  psychiatry at, 223–227
Texas University of San Antonio, 68,
  155, 221–223; curriculum of,
  221–222; graduate and postgraduate education, 223; psychiatric residency training at,
  222, 223
THOMAS, C. S., 115–126, 139
Track system, 47–48
Training. See Psychiatric residency
  training; Psychiatric education
Tufts University, 68
TUPIN, J. P., 174

U

Undergraduate programs, 1–34; at
  McMaster University, 3–18
United Automobile, Aerospace, and
  Agricultural Workers of America, 121, 128; psychiatric benefit plan of, 129–137
University of Arizona, 155, 163–164;
  basic operating philosophy of,
  163; curriculum of, 164; role
  of department of psychiatry
  of, 163–164
University of California, Berkeley,
  130
University of California, Davis, 68,
  150, 155, 173–177; child psychiatry residency training at,
  176–177; medical student education at, 174–175; other
  mental health professional educational programs at, 177;
  residency training at, 175–
  177; role of department of
  psychiatry at, 173–174; student health service at, 176
University of Connecticut, 168–173;
  clerkship of, 170–171; curriculum of, 168–171; elective
  time at, 173; residency training at, 171–173; role of department of psychiatry of,
  168–171
University of Hawaii, 67, 183–186;
  child psychiatry at, 185–186;
  ethnic groups and cultures at,
  185; medical student teaching
  at, 183–184; residency training at, 184–185
University of Hawaii Affiliated Hospital, 184
University of Indonesia, 186
University of Kentucky, 24–25
University of Maryland, 24
University of Minnesota—Duluth,
  193–195; curricular model and
  goals at, 193; objectives of
  medical school at, 193; schematic outline of curriculum
  of, 195
University of Missouri—Kansas City,
  31, 68, 150, 155–156; core
  curriculum at, 196–197; educational plan of school of medicine at, 194, 196; psychiatric
  instruction at, 197–199
University of Nevada—Reno, 202–
  205; community medicine and
  health care at, 204; responsibilities of Division of Behavioral Sciences at, 202–205;
  undergraduate health science
  teaching at, 204–205; undergraduate medical teaching at,
  202–204
University of Oklahoma, 24
University of Oregon Medical School,
  24–25, 33
University of Rochester, 67
University of South Florida, 178–
  183; curriculum of, 179–182;
  development of the College of
  Medicine at, 178; objectives
  of the College of Medicine at,
  178–179; residency curriculum of, 182–183; role of de-

partment of psychiatry of, 180–182

University of Southern California, 24, 68

University of Texas at Austin, 223

University of Texas at Houston, 219–221; organization of educational program at, 219–220; residency program at, 220–221; responsibility of department of psychiatry, 220

V

Veterans Administration, 8, 132–133, 180–181, 199

Videotapes and slide tapes, 8

Viet Nam War, 153

VON MERING, O., 23

W

WARE, J. E., JR., 92

WEBSTER, T. G., 57, 65–70

WEED, L. L., 94

Western Interstate Commission on Higher Education, 36

WILLARD, W., 25

WILLIAMSON, J. W., 94

WOMACK, N. A., 89

Workshop on "Psychiatric Issues in Insurance," 128

World Health Organization of United Nations, 63

Y

YOLLES, S., 21

Z

ZIMET, C. N., 23